bad sex

bad sex

edited by john hoyland

contents

introduction

Conventional wisdom has it that sex is a wonderful experience, and there are countless books and films and TV
programmes and magazines to remind us how wonderful it is
in case we forget.

But sometimes sex isn't so wonderful. Sometimes, in fact,
sex can go hopelessly, maddeningly wrong. This can happen
even if there is no coercion, no abuse. We can want the other
person, or think we do, and have good reasons for thinking
they want us. But then, when we get down to it, sex just doesn't
work out. Instead of making us feel wonderful, it makes us feel
disappointed, used, perplexed, ridiculous, angry, ashamed.

It seemed to me that this was interesting but surprisingly
unexplored territory. Bad sex is something that happens to
almost all of us at one time or another, but we seldom talk
about it, still less write about it – perhaps because the pressure
to be 'successful' in sex is so strong.

Yet experiences of bad sex can be very revealing about
people and how they relate to each other. They can illustrate
the inappropriate perceptions and expectations that people
can bring to their relationships; their capacity for deception
and self-deception; the way their minds and bodies can pull in
different directions; the sheer gulf in understanding that can
exist between them when sex is involved. All in all, few
experiences are so exposing.

This, I thought, was a theme that could inspire some fascinating short stories. Nevertheless, when I started to invite writers to contribute to this book, I had a slight fear that they might want to leave such a subject alone – and indeed, some did. 'Bad sex?' exclaimed one prize-winning novelist. 'I have never experienced any "bad sex", and I wouldn't dream of writing about it if I had!'

In the event, though, I received far more stories than I could possibly include in one book. What's more, people's interpretation of 'bad sex' has been much more varied than I could ever have imagined – to the extent that some of the stories aren't about the physical act of sex at all. Instead, they deal with aspects of our sexual culture that can make people feel bad, or with fears and anxieties about sex that lurk only in the depths of people's minds.

Here, then, are twenty-one tales about a neglected area of human experience: tales of misunderstandings and misadventures; tales of people being used, or denied passion; tales of collisions between fantasy and reality; tales that remind us, as Evelyn Conlon's Michael says, that 'we can't divide the body into sections and make them pretend they have nothing to do with each other'.

Above all, these are stories to be enjoyed – partly because many are funny, partly because many are brave, partly because they tell us much about people that a book about good sex, for example, might well miss.

And partly because there is a particular pleasure in reading them: the feeling that, no matter how many dodgy sexual experiences one may have had oneself, at least it hasn't always been *that* bad.

dear all

kate pullinger

Dear All,

Another year has passed and it's time once again for my annual, up-to-the-minute letter which I send to you all out there. I know some of you feel this is a bit impersonal, but, hey, otherwise you might not hear from me at all. I don't know about you but I really appreciate all the letters I get at Christmas.

Well, it's been quite a year for the Mytel family. Larry and I separated and are filing for divorce. This may seem sudden for most of you, especially if you haven't heard from me since my last Christmas letter. We didn't tell anyone until it was all sewn up. In fact, Larry didn't even tell *me* for a couple of years – he waited until just a few weeks before we put together our separation agreement and best of all, he waited until I had someone in place to fill the gap that his departure would have created. That's where Bob comes in. Larry and I had been friends years ago with Bob and his wife Donna. Bob and Donna have since divorced and while I was at a conference in Toronto I ran into Bob. Over the years Larry often told me that he thought I should be married to Bob, not him. And, when we met again at the conference, Bob also seemed to think he was the perfect man for me and went around the conference cocktail party telling everyone so. I was confused. Where would it all lead? But when Larry started talking 'separation' we both looked to Bob for assistance. And Bob was happy to accommodate us – me. It has all worked out really well. Bob and I are getting married in the spring. Larry has what he wants in his life – to make his own decisions, spend his own money, do his sports, and check out the babes (all the things he wasn't able to do – or rather, wasn't SUPPOSED to be doing while he was with me – because he married so young). And I have what I want in life – a home, a job, and a man who is loving, caring and protective of me. What a good Christmas this is going to be.

Warren continues reading. He hasn't seen Debbie Barnsley – now Debbie Mytel soon to be Debbie someone else – in sixteen years, but he still gets a photocopied letter from her every year, like minutes from the annual general meeting of an alumni society. Warren doesn't send Christmas letters. He likes Christmas, he spends it with his wife and their two kids, but he doesn't send Christmas letters. He receives them though, mostly from old girlfriends like Debbie. He reads them and, as he reads, he remembers things.

Let me tell you about Bob. He and Donna didn't have any kids, so the divorce was straightforward, just like Larry and me. He is six foot four (my mother loves that), 185 pounds, with a head full of beautiful silvery-grey hair – handsome, that's the word I'd use. And I do. Often. He owns one 1965 vintage sports jacket which he inherited from his dad, no dress pants, only jeans, Western shirts, tooled leather belts with big silver buckles, cowboy boots and cowboy hats. Otherwise his wardrobe consists of mountain gear. He has lived in town for twenty years. He's a non-smoker, has given up coffee for over four years now, and seldom drinks.

He's a great cook and loves to have people over for dinner or to stay the weekend. He leaves for work at seven a.m., comes home to fix me lunch (sometimes we don't make it as far as the kitchen), and returns home after six for nice long evenings. And the sex, well, running the risk of sounding crude, let's just say Bob is a *big* improvement on Larry. We stay in a lot, listen to music, cook.

The down side on Bob: he's poor, but of course, he's very happy as I've heard poor people tend to be. He does all the things I find scary and life-threatening but which he and his ilk think of as 'man-stuff' such as horses, guns, motorcycles, and mountains. Sometimes he's so much like Grandpa I can't believe it. He loves to read which is great, but he tends to have read the entire book and remembered the facts of the case and he corrects me when I'm making eloquent sweeping generalizations. Don't ya loathe it! But it really is love. It is wonderful to love and to be so loved. I am so grateful for the opportunity I've been given to live two terrific lives in one lifetime, my life with Larry and now, my life with Bob.

Warren doesn't do 'man-stuff'. He never has. He's surprised to hear Debbie is enjoying that aspect of Bob, she never used to go for macho types. People can change a lot though, especially over the sixteen years since college. Warren himself has changed. He's got two kids for christ's sake, and he loves his wife, and not only at Christmas. He's happy with his job. He sells real estate on Vancouver Island. Debbie wouldn't believe it if she heard that was what he did now. Or perhaps she would. Perhaps even then, when he was a flamboyant and, he thought, Byronic youth, he had the soul of a real estate man.

Bob and I plan to have a family. We're not too old, lots of people have families late these days. We feel very settled together and think that we could give a child a good start in life. We just pray (yes, we *pray* – really, both of us – and it is so wonderful to be with a man with whom I can pray) that we will be able to conceive. Hopefully we will have news for you in our next Christmas letter!

My only other big news is that I've been promoted to senior manager level at work. I've been working on a gigantic project which involves data extrapolation from 2500 files from the Chief Medical Examiner's Office, pulling approximately 1200 suicide notes from those files for analysis. The reasons why people kill themselves are very sad indeed, but I've been down myself and I couldn't say I haven't thought about it once or twice. Haven't we all? Bob says he doesn't want me getting any ideas – and who said he didn't have a sense of humour?!! If there is one thing I miss about Larry, it is the jokes and the laughter. With Bob I am extremely happy, he just doesn't make me laugh so very much. So let's pray for love AND laughter, for us and for everyone of you.

Warren doesn't think he ever met Larry Mytel, he can't quite remember. Nor does he remember Debbie having had a particularly keen sense of humour. Warren isn't much of a joker himself. He likes a laugh, he and his wife Kathy get romantic comedies out from the video store. They have a laugh.

Warren wonders what Debbie's job could possibly be. He thinks he'll find out if Kathy kept Debbie's previous Christmas letters. Maybe if he reads the last decade or so he will be able to figure out where Debbie works. Twelve hundred suicide notes. Phew.

Just then, as Warren sits and stares at Debbie's photocopied letter, Kathy comes into the room.

'What you got there?' she asks.

'Debbie Mytel's Christmas letter.'

'Interesting?'

'Sort of,' says Warren, 'sort of weird. I haven't seen her for sixteen years.'

'Funny how some people like to keep in touch.'

'Yeah,' says Warren. Kathy leaves the room again. She is spending the evening cleaning up after the kids. Once a month she attempts to put everything from all over the house away where it belongs, from where it will levitate over the next month. At the same time Warren is meant to go through all the postal paper work, pay the bills, etc. This is part of their deal. Their relationship is one of many deals – Warren takes the kids to school, Kathy picks them up. Warren babysits while Kathy is at aerobics, Kathy babysits while Warren goes jogging with Al. Warren has sex with Kathy whenever Kathy wants, Warren is always careful to prevent Kathy from conceiving again. Kathy rubs Warren's back when he is tired. They are happy.

Warren would never have been happy with Debbie. Her Christmas letters reassure him of that. They had not been happy even when they were young and had had their – Warren can't bring himself to think of it as an affair and it had been nowhere near as solid as the word relationship suggests – when they were young and had had their . . . thing. It seems such a long time ago. What had they been doing together?

In those days – yes it's true, although Warren can hardly believe it himself – in those days, Warren had thought he might be gay. In fact, he had positively longed to be gay. It had seemed the only way of escaping certain inevitabilities. Warren shakes his head – it turned out that the inevitable wasn't so bad after all. He'd had too much Oscar Wilde too early, that must have been the explanation. He and Debbie had met during their first year at university. Everything seemed wild and strange and confusing. Debbie had developed an enormous crush on Warren. Warren had been bowled over by her. He'd had crushes on other people, plenty of them, all boys. None had ever shown the slightest bit of interest in returning his gaze, but Warren preferred it that way. Debbie was a different proposition. She was smart, she was pretty in a boyish sort of way. She said she didn't care if he was gay, she wanted him anyway. Debbie believed that this made sense and her logic took his breath away. 'Okay,' he said, finally, 'okay'.

They began their evening – that fateful night was how Warren had thought about it even before it happened – in the smoky, beer-soaked bar in the Student Union building. They got rapidly and thickly drunk. They pretended to discuss Immanuel Kant and then they kissed briefly when the time seemed right. Warren thinks he can still remember the taste of Debbie's mouth – beery, he thinks, wet, female. He almost froze then and there, was almost unable to continue. But something pushed him on, led him back to the halls of residence, that something, of course, being Debbie.

Kathy comes back into the room; she is carrying a small bicycle that belongs to their son Teddy. 'What are you doing Warren?' she asks, slightly suspicious.

'Paying the bills,' says Warren, 'they pile up.' Kathy leaves again. Warren looks back down at Debbie's letter.

And so another year has come to an end. I hope all of you out there have a wonderful Christmas, and that you feel as warmed by happiness as Bob and I do. For those of you I haven't seen for a while, well, I've got a few grey hairs now, but nothing a little dye won't cover up!

Happy New Year!

Love Debbie, reads Warren. Warren never did love Debbie. He never had the opportunity after that fateful night. They had gone back to her room. Debbie lit all her candles. She loved candles, they were everywhere. Warren had never had sex with anyone before, he wasn't sure about Debbie. He hoped she knew what she was doing. They sat on the bed, there was only one chair and it was attached to the desk. Debbie put on a record. Abba. Warren asked her to put on something more serious instead, King Crimson or something like that. He felt a bit woozy from the alcohol. Debbie lay down on the bed and closed her eyes. He lay down too, thinking great, we'll just go to sleep, but he quickly realized that wasn't what she meant him to do.

Debbie looked romantic in the candlelight, even more like a boy than usual, a long-haired Edwardian boy. She was giving instructions. One hand here, the other there. Lips. Teeth. Tongues. Even now Warren can remember his fumbling with embarrassing clarity. They began removing different bits of their clothing, sweaters, shoes. He was surprised by her bra, it looked so . . . structural. They pushed their bodies together awkwardly, rubbing this, pressing that. They took off their jeans. Underwear. Everything seemed damp, slippery. Debbie wanted Warren to lie on top of her, so he did, feeling heavy, unwieldy. Debbie had stopped wiggling and was lying very still. She looked up at him, her young face full of expectation, desire and fear. In her eyes he saw their future together, kids, cars, summer holidays. He knew what he was supposed to do next.

'I can't,' he said, rearing back, elbowing Debbie in the stomach, bashing his own head against the wall. 'I don't know why, I just can't.' Warren is speaking out loud now, in his own sitting room.

'Why not?' says Kathy who has returned with another armful of toys. Warren looks up.

'Nothing hon,' he says, embarrassed again. She smiles as she crosses the room.

Later, when he and Debbie had their clothes back on and

were drinking cups of tea, Warren still apologizing and Debbie still on the edge of tears, Debbie had said, 'They have clubs for people like you.'

'What?' said Warren.

'You know, the gay students club, things like that.'

'Oh?' said Warren.

'You don't always have to feel outcast and disgusting.'

'Oh,' says Warren. 'Thanks.'

Kathy comes back into the room. This time her arms are devoid of toys. She comes right up to Warren, plucks Debbie's Christmas letter out of his hands and pushes the dining room table back a foot. Then she places herself unceremoniously on Warren's lap. The weight of her body brings Warren swiftly through the years. He puts his arms around her waist. He remembers that Kathy used to look like a boy, before she had the kids. He says to himself it's not my fault about Debbie and Larry and Bob. Kathy leans back against his chest.

'Maybe we should do a Christmas letter next year,' she says.

'Oh yeah, what would we say?' asks Warren. '"Dear All. Everything is exactly the same this year as it was last year except we're all one year older. We divorced and remarried in the spring. The children share the psychological profile of a serial killer. For those of you who haven't seen me in sixteen years, I've aged well, I now look exactly like Marlon Brando. For those of you that Kathy and I never slept with, well, you don't know what you're missing. Merry Christmas. Love Warren and Kathy."' Warren stops.

'Debbie Mytel,' says Kathy, picking up the letter. 'Did you sleep together?'

'Not really,' says Warren. 'Hardly at all.'

concorde

joseph o'connor

In the shadow of the arches, he looked like the protagonist of a novel. You were so much in love with him that you felt you could fuck him by just thinking about it. You dear sweet man, you thought, as you smiled and said hello, I am completely at your mercy. I cannot tell you what I feel for you because you would laugh and run away and I would not see your heels for dust, my little man, because you would be gone so quickly.

You walked beside him down by the Liffey wall and the air seemed to drone with traffic and blues. The shadows moved across the oily water, shadows of clouds, black shadows of buildings. A tricolour flag was flying from the top of the Custom House. You looked happier than he had ever seen you before.

The suffering look was missing from your face. The haunted raw-boned glance was gone. Your hair was very clean. It smelt clean as lemons and your eyes were wide. You looked heroic, that was what he was thinking. You sat on the wall by Butt Bridge, watching the gulls and the electronic clock. Your eyes were brown as the river. You remember the way he kissed you, the dull throbbing ache of pleasure that seeped down and flowered between your legs. But that is not what he remembers. What he remembers now is the gulls, the cruel sound they made, the rattle of trains, the clock ticking, the stench of the river, the odd light in your brown eyes.

Down by the Harp Bar the night was slinking over frantic soulboys and girls in tight white skirts. You walked up D'Olier Street, past the gates of Trinity. You slipped your hand through his arm and found yourself humming softly, not listening to what he was saying. You ate with him in the Coffee Inn. You had spaghetti, not a good thing to order on a first date. You got it down the front of your shirt. Spaghetti is so democratic that way, he said, and you laughed, although silently, you wondered why. Van Morrison was on the radio, singing 'Madam George'. The clicking clacking of the high-heel shoes.

I would do anything for you, you thought. I would walk into a crowded church and put my hand in the flame of a candle for you.

You said the song always made you sad, although you never really knew what it was about. He started to explain. One of The Waterboys came in, sat at the table next to you. Reading Brendan Behan, scratching his thin, unshaven face. Bright eyes, darting. The kind of eyes that could do a bank robbery. He seemed disappointed that nobody recognized him.

It was the waitress who mentioned it. Midsummer Night, she said. Not that this was any big deal. He was less sentimental than you, or so he insisted. Still, Midsummer Night, he liked the idea of that. It had a certain something. A night for lovers, the waitress said; a marvellous night to fool around and fall in love. You ordered an espresso and stole one of his cigarettes.

The sky over the GPO was a rage of purple and orange, flamelike, exploding above the streets. You saw sailors on O'Connell Bridge, Russian sailors, with white suits and red stars on their caps. They were smoking, laughing at girls, shouting out lines of Irish poetry. They were 'O commemorate me where there is water!' Strolling couples idled past the shopfronts, stealing kisses, almost bleeding with desire. You twined your fingers in his. A thin dirty man with a one string guitar sang 'Blue Moon', under the statue of Jim Larkin. A stone-faced woman with a crucifix wailed Hail Mary's. A traveller girl in a blanket caught your eye and smiled.

You were going to a concert in aid of Nicaragua, or Nicky Kelly, or the ANC, something. It was cancelled when you got there, or over too early, gaggle of disappointed Liberals outside the SFX Centre all desperately trying to be reasonable. The guy from the Socialist Workers Party wouldn't take NO for an answer. You told him no anyway. You told him six quid fifty for a tape of scrawny Albanians singing about their tractors was really a bit optimistic.

No taxi would take you. So you walked with him all the way back down into the hot city and you found a twenty pound note on Gardiner Street. Outside the chapel, where the martyr is buried, the poor man who mortified himself for the sins of Ireland. Blessed Matt Talbot, you said, we have nothing to lose but our chains. Do you remember when you said that? You said it was an omen and he talked about Yeats's face, arrogant as a Roman emperor, there in the middle of the twenty pound note. You told him your mother had it on good authority that Yeats was an awful fucker for the women. You could not throw a stone over a ditch, your mother said, without hitting one of his bastards. You said your mother was great. You never had any problems with your mother, you said.

You walked around for a while, had a couple of beers in some plastic pub thronged with potplants and aspiring novelists. A crowd of black polo-necks sat in the corner yapping about Gabriel García fucking Márquez, how unliterary Roddy Doyle was, how Ivan Klima was just so *Eastern*. You met a friend of his and he latched onto you. He kept looking at your knees. His friend asked you which Greek island was your favourite and you said oh, probably

Catharsis. He hadn't heard of that one. You kicked him under the table and said you both had to go.

You went to a nightclub in the old cathedral. The colours oozed through the stained glass and the bass thundered up through the grating. In the queue you talked about the strange lights in the sky. You said they were shooting stars but he said there was no such thing. You smiled and shook your head. Romantic Ireland's dead and gone, you said. What am I going to do with you?

Inside there were punks on the stairways and accountants on the dancefloor. You can't remember now what you talked about, but you remember looking into his face, watching the way his lips moved, the way he ran his fingers through his hair, the whiteness of his teeth, remember thinking very clearly that this much happiness could not last. You had to lean very close to be heard. He touched your wrist when he spoke to you. The wine tasted cheap and a little too sweet. You didn't dance. He was getting serious.

– Who's looking for a big time thing?, you said, maybe we could just take a chance.

He'd been hurt. Inevitably.

– Sure, go on, you said, take a chance on me, I'm worth it.

He laughed when you told him he was being evasive. Elusive, he said. No, you insisted, that wasn't the same thing at all. You said, Sweet thing, I'd help you with anything. Sweet thing. You did actually say that. You surprised yourself.

Suddenly you stood on O'Connell Bridge at three in the morning, surrounded by sobbing drunkards and Jesus freaks. You ate half a hamburger. You wanted him to take you home. You had your first argument.

The taxi driver told you not to be fighting. Life was too short, he said. And it was summer time, after all. He had a flashing Virgin Mary on the dashboard and a cosh in his glove box. Any trouble, he said, out she comes. Life's too short, he said, for that kind of trouble. The whole city is full of tinkers now, he said, there's not one of them would know the meaning of manners.

You stepped through the door and breathed in deeply. You laughed at the wallpaper and the creepy posters. His flatmate was still awake, listening to that bloody Leonard Cohen record, sunglasses on, icepack on his head, joint the length of a milk bottle jammed into his mouth.

He followed you in and took off his coat, showed you the spare room, all packed up with his dead mother's books. 'The Library' he called it.

– So how's the lovebirds?, flatmate said, is the love train boarding?

– Are they all your books?, you asked him.

– Yeah, flatmate said, he's going into the literature business.

– Goodnight Pete, he said. Flatmate didn't get the drift.

– Goodnight, he said again, a little too firmly.

– Oh, flatmate said, right.

Flatmate picked himself up, raised his slippers to his nose, sniffed them, trailed off to bed, still sucking on the joint.

The sound of the clock seemed very loud, and the birds had already started to sing. You opened the windows to let out the smell of dope.

The bedroom was very small. There was an empty milk bottle on the windowsill. You took off your clothes in the darkness and he started to touch you straight away. He was too quick, because he was not thinking. He opened your jeans like a politician opening a new bridge. You thought about the river, the water in swirls and eddies. He parted your legs and licked you, then looked up at your face like he wanted a medal. He pushed his finger into you, trembling. He kept asking you to tell him how much you liked it. He moved you around. He *arranged* you. He sucked your nipples. He asked you to touch yourself. He wanted to watch you touching yourself. His tongue between your lips tasted of smoke and lager. He called you 'baby'. He kept using euphemisms. He kept using strange harsh words that he must have read somewhere.

He remembers the soft hollow of your shoulder. You remember the shape of his face. When he told you he loved you, you laughed. You held his penis in your hand. It felt hot. You lay down and he pushed into you. Your hands twisted the sheets. He started to cry then. He was crying when he came. He pulled out of you and came over your thighs, then rolled over backwards like a capsizing tanker. You closed your eyes. The river again, water pooling, fish with no eyes. It was a long time ago. He licked his thumb and pushed it into you. It was Midsummer Night, and you were in each other's arms, half-naked, and he was crying, and when you started to come, he put his hand over your mouth because he was afraid that you would wake his flatmate. You did it again, in a variety of efficient positions.

You dreamed of The Beatles playing live at the Hollywood Bowl; white beads of rain slanting down over the silent crowd, John Lennon's breathless sad voice singing a song that you didn't quite recognize. Police sirens wailed down on the dual carriageway. Wind rattled the windowpane.

Next morning you found a book on the floor. *Ulysses*. His dead mother's copy of *Ulysses*. You opened it and began to read out loud. Life begins with the dogs mating in the street, it said. When he was in the kitchen you said you were fed up doing the rounds. He said he was fed up doing the dishes. He sighed.

Please don't say it, you thought. I know you are going to say it, but please just don't. He turned away and looked out at the windowbox. He reminded you that he'd been hurt. As if you didn't know. He had been thinking, he said. It was a mistake, he said. He didn't really think he could get involved just now. He pronounced the word involved as though it was in inverted commas. His therapist didn't think it was a good idea for him to be involved just now.

– So you just wanted your hole, you said.

He turned to you and tried to look disappointed. He put his arms around you and leaned his forehead against your face. Then you looked up through the skylight. And you laughed.

Because just at that moment Concorde was roaring over your heads.

You said it was an omen. It looked vast and white, wings glinting like a crazy bird, lights flashing through the clouds. And it looked like it was moving very slowly, although, of course, it was not. You both stood for what seemed like a long time, looking up through the skylight, until your necks ached, and it was completely gone from view.

– You don't see Concorde over Ireland too much, he said.

Then you sighed. And you pulled away from him. And you told him he was right.

– Yes, you said, maybe there's no such thing as shooting stars after all.

You went to find your watch. He picked up the condoms as discreetly as possible and wrapped them in an old Saturday section of the *Irish Times*. Then he looked at you as though he had never seen you before. As though you were a ghost who had suddenly appeared. When you were dressed, he asked you to hold him, and for some reason you did, and he said he didn't know what was wrong, but he just wanted it to stop.

The carnival was on that day. You both looked like refugees and felt worse. Staggering down Grafton Street, too hot and unshowered, raging thirst and hangover. Rugby players with painted faces throwing beer over each other for charity. Millions of sad-eyed buskers, all doing 'Danny Boy' and 'Moondance'. Suited Mormons handing out books and guilt trips. U2 blaring out of the upstairs windows. Your face was pink. You could still taste him. You could still feel him, pulsing inside you.

You said goodbye at the top of Duke Street. His head was roaring with pain. You said so? and he said he'd give you a call. You told him not to get carried away or anything. What? he said, and his face began to perform. You said you were being sarcastic, and then you kissed his mouth, and the people stared at you as they passed by.

– Say Goodbye to Madam George, you said, and you walked away, without turning around. Turning around would not have been you.

He got a taxi back to his flat and slept for ten hours. The sheets were very cold and they smelt of lemons and come.

You knew one day you would give him back the book. *Ulysses*. You would write something in it. Something about a Midsummer Night's Dream. The end of everything old had happened. This is how people fall in love. You knew that, of course, on your way back home through the crowded streets full of sunlight. The hot pavements blurred but you did not cry. You knew that nothing could ever be the same now. You knew that he was half in love with his hurt, that you could never compete with that. You knew that he wanted to wrap his arms around his hurt and cherish it and slide his tongue into every soft fold of it and fuck it until he was sore and the morning rose up out of the river once again. You knew it now. Yes. The streets were crazy with balloons. You knew what you had done. The knowledge seemed to flood you, move through your body until you were filled with the most unspeakable fear.

strange
attractors

jane delynn

The major sex organ, it is said, is the one between the ears. I prefer to think it is not just the brain itself that is referred to, but the organs of sensation and perception that are lodged in the uppermost part of the body: the eyes, the ear, the nose, the tongue – and others, perhaps, for which there is currently no name.

The events I will be referring to took place long ago, when the cynical idealism of youth had not yet given way to the idealistic cynicism of middle age. I had more energy then, and time, to devote to the amorous arts, and my sexual vanity was naturally not so considerable as it is today. (I use 'vanity' not in the usual pejorative sense of 'vainglorious' or 'excessively proud,' but as regards the very essence of its meaning: 'without real significance or value.') For it was an age when, you see, I still believed in the meaning – both iconographic and 'real' – of those acts of excitement and distress that generally occur between two (but on occasion three or four or even more!) people who find themselves in some way or other – sometimes sexually, but perhaps more often economically or socially – 'attracted' to each other.

I was involved with a woman with whom I had little in common. Our sole shared interest was the theater, for we had met when she had had the starring role in a play I had written – a rather gloomy affair that, although I still include it in my CV,

I would never allow to be shown to an agent. Although her combination of 'vanity' (in the standard sense) and reticence had for some reason driven me wild from the moment I had seen her, and led to tedious and prolonged negotiations with the producer and director over whether or not to 'hire' her – a word I use loosely, for in the downtown theater of those days remuneration tended to be hypothetical rather than actual – she was not particularly effective in the role. But who would have been, given the dialogue she was forced to recite? Have I omitted to mention she was quite beautiful? – delicate, with lovely dark coloring on which a kind of permanent natural blush resided, albeit her brown eyes emanated what to me seemed a rather irritating cow-like placidity.

We were poor then, she even more so than me, and could rarely afford to go to restaurants. Our evenings tended to consist of her cooking me some sort of vegetarian concoction, the consumption of an illegal substance or two (accompanied by, on occasion, a legal one such as beer or wine), and the listening to records, sometimes preceded or succeeded by our attendance at a movie or performance at the kind of inexpensive theater in which my own had first seen the light of – well, night. On occasion we passed the evening in my apartment, but unbeknownst to her my (male, gay) roommate found her company monotonous in the extreme, so generally I created an excuse to stay in hers.

Having little in common (besides which she was not talkative) our conversation consisted almost exclusively of pleasantries concerning plays we had seen or were thinking of seeing, and instruction as to how to properly prepare vegetables. For variety we discussed yoga, which she practiced and I pretended I wanted to. The rest of the time, we were either silent, or I, the Writer, held forth, sometimes on my current *kvetches* and sometimes on my childhood. (Sometimes, these were the same.) In spite/because of the tedium of conversation and the ritual predictability of our encounters, I loved her madly.

Because she meditated, because she practiced yoga, because she abjured the incensing effects of meat, I could never decide whether her conversational reticence was due to some flaw such as shyness or lack of intelligence (or, at least, quick-wittedness), or was, conversely, evidence of some profounder wisdom having to do with the pointlessness of speech and the 'vanity' (in *my* sense) of all endeavor. When on occasion I made inquiries into the causality of her serenity, she would inevitably remain motionless for several minutes, then a peculiar smile would pass across her face, her nostrils would dilate, and she'd give a beatific shrug. It was a response identical in spirit (and almost so in appearance) to her inevitable response of 'nothing' when I would interrogate her as to what she was thinking.

In those days I thought I knew everything – not just about the world but about myself and other people, including thoughts and feelings that supposedly resided in the unconscious – so I rarely took people at their word, but would probe beneath surface speech and actions for the hidden meaning I was sure I could somehow divine. My next-to-most recent therapist ascribed such attitudes to 'grandiosity,' but I think it had more to do with boredom. When I did not find the world (rather, that particular part of it on which I was currently bestowing my attention) worthy of my interest, I would simply invent the sub-text to make it so. Indeed, is not Love the invention of a sub-text so coherent, persuasive, and enthralling that, on occasion, the narrative it creates so overpowers the apparent commonsensical one that no amount of contrary or even contradictory 'real world evidence' can have the slightest a/effect on its shape? Thus, when Mirabelle (for such was her name) replied 'I don't know' to a question of whether Presidents Kennedy, Johnson, or Nixon would be judged by God (should S/He exist) most culpable in relation to the Vietnamese (against whom our war had only recently *officially* ended), I did not even consider accepting this reply at face value – as a simple acknowledgment of insufficient confidence in her knowledge and/or judgment – but fabricated in my mind an unspoken monologue which provided a resonant and intellectually worthy explanation for her only *apparently* vapid and non-committal utterance, as well as giving a sympathetic and morally admirable reason for not disclosing such explanation to me: the well-intentioned (but – on some deep level – profoundly naive) questioner.

It is hard to recreate such internal monologues, but to the best of my recollection this one ran something as following:

'Johnson and Nixon are mass murderers . . . everybody knows that.

'She threw Kennedy in there to irritate me – knowing I and everybody else like him – we have discussed this before and what would be the point of hashing it through again?

'In such instances of villainy, which of the two is worse hardly matters – nor do I believe she thinks it matters. She just wants to argue with me no matter whom I pick.

'Because I see no point in arguing, I'll reply "I don't know," rather than telling her there is no point to her question, for although she surely knows it herself, my articulation of it will hurt her, she is so sensitive. After all, is it not better for me to look "stupid" than her, since my ego is so much less invested in intelligence than hers?'

On the night in question we had gone to an inexpensive play in an East Village theater in which the actors were paid by the sharing of the gate receipts – an amount that one could not even count on to cover the requisite post-performance repast. It was a play in which, as was common in those days (as in ours

– not to mention Shakespeare's) male actors assumed female roles. At the time I was more excited by the nuances of gender confusion than feminism, so the logical corollary – why were women not assuming the roles of men? – did not occur to me. I had, in short, enjoyed the play, and so, to all appearance, had Mirabelle.

We bought some beer and climbed the steps to her sixth-floor apartment. Her building was in the heart of the old Greenwich Village, and, by dint of the fortuitous placement of nearby buildings, commanded a clear view of surrounding rooftops and a sliver of the Hudson. This night, with perhaps a quarter moon, you could discern, if you squinted your eyes, whitecaps on the river; several blocks south a crowded and brightly illuminated rooftop gave strong indication that a movie was being shot. Inexplicably (and therefore tantalizingly), the set consisted of a little wooden house, several café tables and an old-fashioned telephone booth.

We sat in our usual silence while watching the proceedings, then of a sudden the bright lights dimmed, taking with them, so I felt, a bit of the magic of the evening. Mirabelle must have experienced something similar, for almost immediately she got up and asked if I would like her to put on some music, which until that moment we had managed to do without.

'Please.'

She squatted on her knees, pawing through the records till she found some Keith Jarrett, who served the function then that New Age music would later in the decade. 'Would you like another beer?'

'Sure,' I said. But she did not take another for herself, so I sipped mine very slowly. I would have pounded the top back on the bottle would that not have looked like I could not make a decision for myself.

I talked for awhile about the play itself, and then the acting (which – having been trained in some watered-down version of The Method – she denounced for focusing too much on such 'surface-y externals' as vocal intonation and bodily gesture), then she went into the bedroom and came out with a little wooden box which contained illegal but nonetheless relatively inexpensive products of the hemp plant. Sitting on the floor beside the coffee table, she spread out a piece of paper and began sifting out the dried-up flowers from the seeds and twigs. She was frugal and always performed this part of the operation slowly and delicately, whereas I, less conscientious and meticulous, would invariably lose patience, and end up with little sticks poking their way through the papers of my joints.

When she was done, she placed a single sheet of the white rolling paper on the table, then carefully sprinkled a thin and even line of the herb across it. After smoothing out this row, and winding the paper in a tight little cylinder so that it would burn slowly and evenly, having twisted one end closed and the other somewhat less so (so as to allow sufficient passage of air to maintain combustion), she placed just enough saliva on the yellow glue strip to ensure the seal would hold, while nonetheless allowing the paper to remain sufficiently and miraculously dry. Mine inevitably dissolved into a soggy mess that was not just esthetically unpleasant but created almost insurmountable difficulties in both lighting and sustained smoking.

Although with insufficient patience to roll an adequate joint myself, I somehow always possessed more than enough to cheerfully witness these slow and somewhat self-absorbed preparations.

'Here,' she said, extending the exquisitely-made object to me. She always offered me the first hit, and for some reason this ceremonial politeness never failed to enchant me. Although smoking marijuana in large groups often made me nervous, and could unnerve me even in her presence, I always forced myself to accompany her in her ingestion of the various stimulants and relaxants and hallucinogens, for fear that we would no longer be able to converse at all if our bodies were not being affected by the same constituency of chemicals.

'Thanks.'

She struck a match and leaned over. The light isolated and made even more striking the angles of her cheekbones. Then the end of the cigarette began to glow red, and I tried to stifle a cough.

After several hits, I handed the joint to her. She inhaled, then leaned her head against the base of the couch and shut her eyes. The cigarette dangled from her fingers, but due to the skill with which she had rolled it, it neither died out nor consumed itself. It made me nervous hanging there, but I dared not remove it from her fingers lest she think I was trying to censor her activities.

The slow dilation of her nostrils provided the only indication she was alive. As usual, it was impossible to tell if she were asleep or merely ruminating. The question of which, irrelevant though it might prove to the objective correlatives, was of immense import to me, providing a framework, as it were, for my creation of the sub-text. That is, as long as I continued to believe she was in a meditative state my brain would continue its invention of her internal monologue, but such narration would immediately cease were I to determine she was sleeping. This, in turn, would cause me to become both bored and irritated, both because I would have nothing to fill my mind and because of the consequent likelihood that our sexual activities would be curtailed or even eliminated.

Perhaps this is the place to interject that, not considering herself truly one of the tribe that prefers women (and, indeed, being embarrassed to the point of concealment by such relations with me), my endeavors towards her in that direction were generally far more abbreviated and constrained than they would have been with someone who did not dispute the propriety of such actions. This should not imply, however, that I did not enjoy sex with her. On the contrary, I enjoyed it all the more due to its unpredictable character. Even the lack of passion (indeed, *distaste*) with which she on occasion stroked my body had ceased to disturb me, for this very apathy – by eliminating the self-consciousness I tended to feel concerning the intensity of my reactions – tended to relax and soothe me, thereby making it easier to achieve the magnitude of response that so often eluded me in the presence of those possessing greater expertise and fervor.

To put it another way, the reflexive perversity of my reactions – my unconscious inability to acquiesce to another's desire to arouse me – lost its compulsive quality in the presence of her indifference, and for perhaps the first time in my life I was able to sexually respond to someone in a relatively straightforward, unstylized fashion.

So when I asked her what she was thinking, it was not because I had reason to expect any answer other than the usual, but because I was anxious to determine the degree of her alertness. To be sure, I was aware of the tenuousness of the approach; sometimes even when she was awake she would choose not to reply to what (after all) seemed to her my redundant inquiries.

'I was trying to remember the words of this song.'

'What song?'

'The one I'm supposed to perform at the audition tomorrow.'

'I didn't know you had an audition.' This news upset me, for she was particularly anxious about her sleep before such appearances. 'Would you play it for me?'

'You'd like to hear it?' she asked, with surprise, as if anything that concerned her had ever not interested me.

'Of course.'

She pushed herself to her feet and walked over to the spinet.

On it were piled songbooks and on top of these sheet music, which in the dark (the room was illuminated only by two candles) she was compelled to flip through slowly.

As I studied her profile my heart caught with her beauty, and it seemed that, despite the remarks of my roommate, nothing else would ever matter. She sang in a mezzo-soprano with vibrato and often came in a bit late on her notes – for which 'cheapness' of effects my roommate had nothing but the most disparaging comments, even as he (somewhat paradoxically, I felt) refused to concede even the intensionality of such adornments.

After several songs she yawned. Although I enjoyed her singing, I was not distressed at this allusion to slumber. After she had emerged from the bathroom, I quickly brushed my teeth and washed my face, then stripped off my clothes and hopped into bed. She, as usual, remained at her little dressing table, performing the various rituals relating to the removal of makeup and the subsequent application of various night-time conditioning and replenishing lotions. My enjoyment of this – like the rolling of the cigarettes and the discussions about vegetables – never palled. Indeed, though surely part of my interest was due to anticipation of the further possibilities of the evening, I have always enjoyed observing the ablutions and repairments of women – both ones I was involved with and others whom I saw in public toilettes during intermissions of sundry artistic events – perhaps (as my previous therapist but two suggested), either because I used to observe my mother doing so, or because I did *not*.

'Love': what is it about? Is it an affliction of the flesh or the soul, or a confluence of the two? Is it a blessing or a curse, or both together? Is it the very personification of the human tendency to waste time – or, conversely, the only activity worth pursuing? How often did I ponder such notions as I watched her, how rarely could I decide the proper answer!

Bored as I often was in her presence, how much more so was I in her absence! Perhaps, as my roommate complained, there was no 'there there.' Perchance, as my roommate contended, the true locus of her existence was only in my imagination. Quite possibly, as my roommate proclaimed, I had invented her not so much to ward off the Void (as I grandiosely told myself), but because I had lost confidence in my ability to attract someone with greater internal resources.

Even were this all true, I did not care. Her quietness, her coldness, her lack of enthusiasm, served as proxies for my own deficiences in such arenas, and enabled me, conversely, to feel optimistic, enthused, alive.

When she had finished with the dressing table she turned out the light and delicately climbed into bed, where she lay with her back towards me as near the edge as possible. I was used to this and did not mind, though initially it had bothered me. But I had overcome my reluctance at *her* reluctance when I discovered that it could usually be overcome by a show of interest and persistence on my part. 'Come here,' I said, after I had sidled over to her and placed my hand on her side.

She turned towards me with that weird shrug and a smile. In the dark we stared at each other. I told myself these were the eyes of a tiger, not a cow. I pulled her to me and, very slowly, as if she were a most delicate doll, as if nothing could be more gross than sticking a tongue in another person's mouth, rested my lips lightly on hers.

A long while later, for I broached each new position as delicately as a spy, as surreptitiously as if I were a teenage boy in a movie theater pretending to watch the film even as he fumbles to unhook the bra with a single hand, I found myself lying, my head a little raised, near the foot of the bed, with Mirabelle's legs spread in a curling V or U around my neck, her eyes closed and the emblem of a smile (rather than a smile itself) across her lips. She was breathing shallowly but rapidly as I moved my tongue back and forth, then in a counterclock-wise circle, initially at low speed and intensity, with an intermittent and casual flick, like the languid exploration of a sleepy snake. And occasionally, for demi-seconds, I did fall asleep, waking with a guilty start which – had our positions been reversed – I would have instantly recognized by the increase in pressure and speed with which that newly-awoken tongue attacked my body, but which change of motion she never seemed to notice. As the minutes transpired I would gradually increase either the speed or the intensity of these motions of my tongue – not so slowly that the conception of progression would utterly disappear from her consciousness, yet slowly enough that the narratives of titillation and frustration, of resistance and submission, could not fail to be – at least in some subliminal fashion – present in her mind. Then on occasion, for brief milliseconds of time, at (and this is most important!) *randomly*-placed intervals – I would cease action altogether, lest the pattern of titillation itself become predictable and, hence, *un*titillating.

In short, there was a conscious structure to my labors, and I worked as hard and thoughtfully at my calling as I did on my scripts, to ensure that the climax would be as intense and thrilling, as unexpected and yet (in retrospect) as dramatically necessary as any play's. My basic strategy, you might say (though of course this was an improvisational art, subject to vicissitudes of mood, moon phase, amount and quality of recent encounters, and the degree of artificial stimulants and relaxants in both our bodies) was to insinuate the notion of 'timelessness' by a slow and consistent pace, for the purpose of creating in Mirabelle's mind a belief that whatever was happening would (in some sense) continue 'forever' (i.e. as long as was necessary), at which point, having alleviated temporal anxiety as to untimely cessation – for surely nothing upsets the delicate balance of orgasm so much as the concept of being rushed (except when, on occasion, it functions in the very opposite fashion!) – I would commence the introduction, by the afore-mentioned increases in speed or pressure, of the concepts of teleology and finality – hence death – and it was this dialectic of time vs. eternity, of excitement vs. stasis, of epiphanic enlightenment versus innate knowing, that was responsible (I believe) for the extraordinary intensity of the reaction not just of Mirabelle, but (there is no point in being unduly modest!) of virtually everyone who has come in intimate contact with my tongue.

It is unnecessary, of course, to go into detail concerning the standard 'objective correlatives' – heavy breathing, redness of facial skin, 'involuntary' movements and sounds, outpour-ings of sweat, convulsive graspings of my head and back – which are the inevitable (and, when you think of it, rather frightening and repellent) accompaniments to the gaining of such knowledge, and perhaps I should add that I was not wholly averse to the usage of such 'surfacey' externals as melodramatically bucking my body or mimicking my partner's breathing patterns, not unlike the acting style of the theatrical group we had seen earlier in the evening. This served the dual purpose of convincing Mirabelle that we were undergoing analogous experiences (thereby contributing to the -- perhaps subliminal – narrative of 'unity') and also, by means of this mimickry, to at least partially *achieve* this unity – on the level of heartbeat and breath, at least, if not of one's innermost *soul*. To be a good lover, I have often said, is to use your ears correctly!

But sometimes, though I did my best to imitate a partner, she would not issue her clues correctly, would insist on breathing faster than her internal state would really justify (possibly in the attempt to create some narrative of her own – such as 'call girl' or 'class slut'), and I would have to slow down and re-start, as it were, the entire scenario. Not that one can precisely re-start it – no more than one can duplicate on one night the rhythms and gestures of another – but by changing my pace and activities I would implant, let us say, the notion of 'intermission' in my partner, so that the lack of early fulfillment could be interpreted not as 'failure' (on *either* of our parts), but rather as something inherent to the structure of this particular interaction, something planned, as it were, rather than accidental. And the creation of a belief in the 'purposeful-ness' of the interaction would resonate with the earlier notion of 'timelessness' so as to transform the self-conscious anxiety-producing question of *whether* one would reach epiphanic fulfillment into the more benign (and curiosity-inducing) one of *in which particular manner* on this particular night would this particular dramatic crisis be resolved.

To put it another way, you might say that I had switched the genre from mystery to that of suspense. And with the return of this rather detached curiosity, there would be room for Eros to creep back in. The particular method of the *intermezzo* might include such *divertimenti* as the licking of the back of the knee, or the massaging of a gum with my tongue, or pulling of hairs from the pubic area in my teeth – anything that would allow us to re-order our breathing and re-group our resources before recommencing the tedious work. For tedious work it some-times is when (let's not beat about the bush!), exhausted and (therefore) lacking in imaginative resources, one must ani-mate what may momentarily seem like a piece of wiry brillo with the luster and passion of a human being and all its wishes, thoughts, fears, and desires . . . when, to be honest, what may be filling the soul is disgust and revulsion.

I use the words 'disgust' and 'revulsion,' but these are of course secondary emotions laid, as it were, over the more humanist ones of desire and triumph with which the sex act is hopefully accompanied. I am a 'sensualist,' yes, but how much is ordinarily left out of our concept of this word – for is not every lowering of face onto an unknown and untested torso as much a leap of faith into the dark as that of a body into a lake at night, with its possibilities of foul smells, hidden protuberances, and unexpected denizens, not to mention incompatibility of pheromones or rhythms, phobias and fetishes, from all of which there is no turning back – at least if one has been brought up in such a way as to possess the standard quota of good manners?

Possessing such – for better or worse – I invariably felt honor-bound to persist in my task until satisfied hands clutched my hair to the breasts (my head following), the digits gently touching my face and arms and back until moans soften and the tortured breaths of satisfaction become half-snores, or – on the rare occasion – in despair push my fingers from the hopeless task. I believe in such sad moments it is I rather than my partner who experiences the greater distress, for the disheartening sense of failure and guilt, combined with empathy for the unsatisfied and disgruntled state, so evokes in me the utter pointlessness of human endeavor, the utter frailty of human connection and the impossibility of Love, that I become peculiarly undone, and, smitten by the utter vanity of existence, lie almost Lifeless until, miraculously, some such external intrusion as the telephone or the emergence from cloud cover of the sun occurs to make the quiescent reptile active once again . . . pointless, pointless, pointless!

To return to Mirabelle. This particular night, I vowed, would be special. This particular night we would attain heights of bliss as yet unequaled in our (well, really *my*) exertions. This particular night she would be driven to such extremes that those fearsome words – 'I love you' – would emerge, undesired but unsuppressible, from her lips. And with the utterance of these magic totems, our relationship would be transformed – the sub-text articulated, the narrative conceded – and she would clasp my arm, chattering gaily, oblivious to all onlookers, as we sauntered carefree down the street. And courtesy of this unharnessed wit, courtesy of the freedom with which she could share all her little secrets with me, her love in turn would flourish, and multiply . . . etcetera.

With such hopes I commenced my efforts, with such hopes I found her legs forming a V or U around my neck, breathing shallowly but rapidly as I moved my tongue back and forth, then in a counterclockwise circle, faster and faster, with occasional demi-seconds of cessation to mix hope with fear, to create a correlative in her mind for the *frissons* of her body, to show her there was nothing – no thought, no movement, no emotion – that I could not affect as I chose. And she came along with me, she was my slave as much as (in another sense) I was hers; I was a musician on her body, the slightest twitch of my fingers or tongue evidenced their immediate effects on her vocal register, her muscle tremors, the emanation of her bodily fluids. And just when she had thought she had reached the apogee, when the waters of her river were about to run into the sea, when the mystery was about to be revealed, the culprit unmasked, I began, ever-so-slightly, to slow down. And though you may think this a crass attempt to conclusively demonstrate to her once and for all the utter dependence of her every flush, her every drop of sweat upon my whims, the truth of it was another matter entirely: we had reached a place where we had never been.

I have mentioned the concept of 'timelessness' before, I believe, but then it was as one-half of the dialectic – one element in the great Western dualities of Life vs. Death, Action vs. Passivity, Diversity vs. Unity, etc. But as our heartbeats slowed in unison, as our breaths began to flatten and smooth, we approached, in the evenness of inhalation and exhalation, via the glacial pace of meditation, that place where not just Time but its opposite (and the duality this represented – 'Time vs. Timelessness') disappeared, where the

Many did not just become One but where Distinction itself vanished. In short, we had reached a place beyond words, beyond thought, a site where desire and fear, past and future, had no meaning, a locus necessarily devoid of artificial tensions and such cheap dramatic compulsions as climaxes and denouements, a zone without boundary or dimension in which we rode forever at the speed of light on a beam of particles or waves – take your pick! – towards an ageless, soundless, eternal present.

I had never been so *there* with anyone. I licked, not her skin, but the hairs of her skin. I blew on them like the wind moving across grass, and my hairs rose and fell with hers because the wind struck me too, and when I inhaled so did she, Siamese linked at the lungs . . . No, we were closer than that, not just twins but mirror images, identical beings occupying the same place at the same time, unperceived as con-terminous due only to the epistemological limitations of a three-dimensional universe. And because I was her, I breathed her slow, calm, constant, evenly-spaced breaths, and I knew, had I been in the realm of the dialectic, the dramatic unities would have been revealed as they never had before.

If it was true for me, by definition it was true for her.

A deep peace ran through me/us, and I felt I/we knew everything. I/we lay there immobile for a few minutes, basking, then I realized my arm, where my head was propped, was aching badly.

I needed to move it. But if I moved it, would I not recall her to the world of 'I' and 'you,' of passion and pain, of things that gush and throats that utter superficial (albeit pleasurable) cries of joy?

It would. Because I loved her, because we lie to those we love, because we lie to ourselves to preserve our love, I tried to distract her/me by altering the movements of my tongue. But this was merely a mechanical diversion. I could not stop thinking of my arm and how, if I did not change position soon, circulation would stop completely and I would develop gangrene.

An honest person – a person who would have been willing to admit the evanescence of all that was and is and is to be – would have simply rearranged her limbs. But I continued the charade of Oneness and Unity as by the tiniest of (hopefully indiscernible) increments I ever so slowly and uncomfortably maneuvered myself off one arm and onto the other.

These exertions fatigued me, and I began to breathe more quickly. To my surprise she did not match my increased pace, but maintained the slow and constant rhythm of her in- and exhalations, even when (so as to distract her from these breathing changes) I further varied the speed and pressure of my tongue.

Her continued indifference to these fluctuations, demonstrating as it did how thoroughly estranged we had become, so upset me that I knew my only hope of vanquishing my sorrow was by sharing it with her. Thus, in search of the comfort of speech, her breath on my neck, the dab of her tongue against the corner of my lip, I began to inch my way up her body.

But even in the face of this desperate journey she managed to maintain composure. When I lay my head next to hers, when I flicked the tip of her nipple with my reptilian tongue, her steady breathing did not alter in the slightest, save for the slight increase in amplitude of a certain sound, which readily could have been explained by my closer proximity to its source. This noise, which accompanied each inhalation and exhalation, I initially could not identify, familiar though it was, but as I drew ever nearer her lips it became ever more distinct and, somehow, disturbing, reminding me of . . . something . . . on the tip of my tongue . . .

A snore! She was sleeping. Had been sleeping, perhaps, throughout our entire surf ride on the perfect wave.

The defining moments in a person's life are few. Until that moment I had somehow – despite a vast preponderance of evidence to the contrary – managed to preserve the conviction that, given world enough and time (i.e. sufficient energy on my part and the merest tendency towards reciprocity on someone else's) there was no one in the universe whose will could prove resistant to my desires. I had felt that, in some fashion, I knew *everything*, that mere closing of lips and the shutting of eyes were but insufficient barriers to my gnostic infiltrations, that when I lay face to torso with another, the secrets of the Universe would be revealed. If not all-powerful, I was surely omniscient, and what was the sub-text, the narrative I was continually inventing, but the on-going Bible of my world?

Mirabelle's snore, with its irrefutable demonstration of the vanity of my beliefs, the narcissism of my imaginings, the absurdity of my longings, was a concrete refutation of all I had held dear. No Loss of Dialectic, no Oneness, no Conquering of Time; we were neither musician nor slave, but a foolish writer and a tired actress. All we were sharing – perhaps all we had ever shared – was a bed!

And as the force of these revelations sunk into my exhausted brain (for such inventions are the hardest of work!) my Love began to die, so that by the next morning when Mirabelle poured my tea I was as irritable and bored as even my roommate could have desired me to be, and I rushed home to tell him how right he had been to advise me not to waste so much time and energy on one who was so clearly not worthy of my passion.

beasts

lisa appignanesi

Women's hair has grown longer again. It sweeps over
shoulders, covers the back of necks. Robert can't remember
when he last saw so little neck and so much hair. Fifteen years,
twenty perhaps. And he is an expert on the backs of women's
heads.

On the plane which had brought him to London, he had
skimmed an article which announced the vulnerable look.
Flowing little girl hair, downcast eyes, pale pouting mouths,
flowery frocks. Just as it was then, but different. The
difference, he imagines, is only partly in him.

Robert Bates shifts his perch on the book-heaped table. It
creaks uneasily and one of the volumes falls to the floor. As he
stoops to pick it up, a woman sitting in front of him turns to
glare at him. Her eyes are fierce, despite the supposed
vulnerability of the hair.

It's okay, he wants to tell her, It's my wife's book. She won't
mind. But, of course, he doesn't say it. And in any case the
curtain of hair has already fallen back into place. It comes to
him, now that the fashion has passed, that he used to like those
bared necks. You could read a character from their lines, their
smoothness, their colour, shape and set, even a certain
vulnerability. Two or three square inches of flesh that didn't
have to pass the morning mirror test. The last terrain of un-
self-consciousness. Secret to the bearer.

Robert doesn't dare sit down again, though he does put his wife's book back on the pile. *Secret Pleasures*. It is *Secret Pleasures* that has brought him here to this crowded upstairs room of a bookshop where tables have been shifted to accommodate as many uncomfortable brown chairs as possible and where the air has grown stuffy with the yearning of too many bodies. This week it is London, but he has been in many spaces like this before, bigger and smaller, in Rome and Paris and Stockholm and Boston and New York, though he won't go West. Every two years or so, every time a new book by his wife appears, he renews his expertise in the backs of heads, mostly female.

Other expertises are his, of course. At home in Connecticut, he is an expert in divorce law. Then he watches people's faces, sees lips curl in lies, eyes flash in rage and greed, the contortions of resentment. When he stands to argue a case in the courtrooms of his native state, it is the back of *his* head which is on display. He likes to veer round quickly to see whether he can catch anyone in the act.

From the tensed forward thrust of the ranked shoulders and the growing dampness in the massed air, Robert can tell that Yvonne has now done away with pleasantries and reached the point in her talk where the secret pleasures speak their name. In public. He tunes in to her voice. It is a cool, even voice, reassuring without being clinical or intimate. It reminds him of the voice of a childhood librarian. It used to thrill him that she could talk dirty in that cool precise voice. Now he wonders whether the thrill had less to do with the dirt than with the excitement of a secret intimately shared.

Even from this distance, he can see how her well-formed lips purse slightly as she speaks the word he least likes . . .

'Masturbate. The pleasures of masturbation for women, the security of . . .'

Her eyes search him out as the sentence rolls on. Robert

smiles that slow encouraging smile he knows she likes and ceases to listen. The matter of Yvonne's talk is hardly new to him. He has read this book, like all her others, in several versions. He also knows that their eyes having once met, she won't seek him out again. What he knows less well is why this particular book has the power to make him feel queasy. He disapproves of it and disapproves of his disapproval. He is a man who is used to admiring his wife.

To reach the stairs Robert has to squeeze his way past the drinks table and a gaggle of late-comers. He tries to do this as inostensibly as is possible for a man of six-foot-two in a summer suit which is too white in the book-darkened space. He senses glares again and is tempted to glare back.

Outside, though a glance at his watch tells him it is already seven-fifteen, the light is so bright he reaches into his pocket for sunglasses. After the stuffiness of the crowded room, the air feels fresh. Robert breathes deeply, relishing even the car fumes.

Behind the sunglasses, he can ponder again why that word so troubles him. It is not the simple act itself. He has no difficulty with that in the abstract or the concrete. Or does he? Perhaps it is just that ridiculous coincidence of a name. He can still vividly remember the humiliating moment in his twelfth year when a boy who had just come back from England had begun to taunt him in the school yard and shout for everyone to hear, 'Master Bates, Master Bates,' and before Robert had quite realized what was up everyone was staring at him, hooting. Luckily he had gone off to high school soon after that.

The street is a climbing one with a village prettiness. There is a clocktower almost at its crest. Robert walks towards it and then turns into a narrower winding street, crossing over when he starts to puff to walk down the other side. That morning, in the strange largeness of the hotel room mirror, he had noticed that his salt and pepper hair had lost most of its pepper. He commented on it to Yvonne, and she told him in her matter-of-fact way that it made him look all the more distinguished. She added, a little ruefully, that if the tables were turned, she would look extinguished.

It was nonsense. Apart from a few lines around her eyes and a slight thickening beneath the shoulder blades, Yvonne has hardly changed in all the years of their marriage, except for the better. His case is different.

Though Robert doesn't like to think about it too often, he knows that this last book of hers has foisted him into a midlife crisis. It is not a crisis of the usual kind. He can still get it up, even for his famous wife, and he has no particular desire to get it up for anyone else with short or long hair. All that is in the past.

No, the crisis is about something else. He has half-decided that this latest book of hers has only served to reveal it to him. It has alerted him to how much times have changed. He cannot hold that against her, though he does. It feels to him as if she has joined the enemy. He is a little confused about it, but this is what he thinks he sees.

When they were both young, back in the late sixties, they believed in openness. Sex had to be named and lived for what it was, guilty secrets bared, the shrouds of hypocrisy rent so that a passionate or playful freedom could breathe and romp. It all seemed so innocent now. Yvonne had gone on the woman's trail and he had backed her in that. After all, how could men be free if women weren't? He had loved her books which plumbed women's travails with mothers and sisters and men and charted their fantasies as lucidly as a Princesse de Clèves drawing a map of love.

And then, he couldn't quite put his finger on when the change had begun, everything had shifted. It was as if they had set off for a picnic on a warm spring afternoon on a motor scooter. The wind played through their hair. Her arms were warm around his waist. But somewhere along the road, the scooter had been transformed into a powerful motorbike and they were driving fast, too fast, careering wildly, she in front. Soon they acquired the garb to go with the bike, policeman's helmets, truncheons, guns, the tools of control and coercion. So that by the time they reached the picnic ground, it had vanished to be replaced by a fenced exercise yard, patrolled by vigilant guards. There were sets of rules and orders and prescriptions for every movement of hands and voice and lips and psyche.

The sexual play of the sexes, Robert grieves, has become a matter of legislation and fixed penalties. It is not so much that he has a nostalgia for the past. He only wishes that the present were other.

Robert isn't happy with the image his mind has presented to him. But then, despite the clarity of the light and the charm of the street, he isn't a happy man. He stops in front of a newsagent's and scans a rack of foreign papers. The headlines tell him in a variety of languages that the world is a mess. The world is a mess and he is worrying about the fact that his wife has written a book about masturbation which tells you to do it and how. In bed, in the shower, on the telephone, to music, to fantasy, or to another's voice, for maximum pleasure and maximum safety. Alone or together. The last worries him. As a lawyer, he wonders whether doing it together can technically stand up as masturbation. But that is a semantic quibble.

On a whim Robert picks out a copy of *Le Monde* and goes into the shop. There is a young woman behind the counter at the far end, beyond the sweets and picture cards and magazines. She has short bristling hair and mulberry lips. A dangling feather earring casts a shadow on her cheek. Fashion has forgotten her. Robert smiles.

The young woman looks up and through him and continues

to flick the pages of her glossy with nails that match her lips. His distinguished hair renders him invisible, Robert thinks. With a slight scowl, he turns towards the magazine shelves. He is surprised by a row of airbrushed female flesh on display in a variety of provocative postures. A perfect bottom sits just above his distinguished hair.

At random, he picks out three of the magazines, plus a copy of *The Economist* and the *London Review of Books*. He puts the porn under his more respectable selections and places the whole lot on the counter in front of the young woman. Robert waits for her reaction.

She taps out the prices on the cash register slowly, but she doesn't pause or blink when she comes to the porn, even when her mulberry nail in search of a tiny number skates over a heavy bosom.

'That's £12.90,' she announces in a bland nasal voice.

Robert is disappointed. Given her appearance, he had expected at least surprise, would have preferred that condemnatory glower which named him a beast. He has forgotten that he is in England, half-way to Europe after all. This thought lifts his spirits.

'Thank you very much,' Robert gives her his charming, open smile. But she has already turned to the next customer and he is left to tuck his offending bundle into the flimsy pages of *Le Monde*.

The act so engrosses him that he is startled by the sound of a 'Hello'. A naked woman straddling a motorbike slips to the ground as Robert looks in the direction of the greeting.

'I saw you leaving the talk. In the bookshop. Over the road.'

The speaker is a slender woman with dark suitably long hair and chocolate eyes. As Robert stoops to pick up his magazine, he mumbles an 'Oh', and adds, once he has regained his height, 'Is it finished?'

She shakes her head, but her gaze is on the magazine in

Robert's hand. She lifts an eyebrow. 'Quick conversion to the cause, or are you rushing off to do it?'

For a moment Robert doesn't know what she means. Then he can't tell whether she is disapproving or merely laughing at him. There is a slight purr of Irish in her voice. She has the face of one of those Paris street urchins with eyes too large and nose too small for real beauty. But he likes the cheekiness of her expression.

'Neither. Just a little impulse shopping.' Robert surprises himself with his own honesty. 'I haven't had an impulse like it for years,' he confides.

'Really?' Her eyebrow rises another notch and this time she bursts into laughter.

They have reached the street now and Robert wishes there were still enough sun to warrant sunglasses. But there isn't. There is, however, a café just to their right, and emboldened by the sound of her laughter, Robert asks, 'Would you like a drink? I'm waiting for someone to come out.' He gestures towards the bookshop.

'Why not? I'm waiting too.'

Robert is pleased by her answer. In America, even without the offensive magazines under his arm, he wouldn't dare ask a woman inside or out of his wife's lectures, to have a drink with him. Increasingly it seems to him that when the massed ranks of the women look at him to see him, their gazes are filled with hostility. Men have been turned into beasts. At their best, they are simply germridden unfeeling beasts, insensitive to women's pleasure. At their worst, they are rampaging, raping, marauding, polluting beasts.

It is not that Robert doesn't know that men, particularly in groups under the direction of a leader, are capable of gross beastliness. It is simply that he knows that all men aren't always and ever beasts. And whereas he used, without thinking, to think of himself as a human being, he is now forced to think of himself as only a testosterone driven male animal. Robert's level of testosterone has not for a long time now, if ever, produced frenzy. Of late, it seems only to produce philosophical ruminations of a depressing kind. As a result, he no longer knows how to think of himself at all.

So Robert is grateful to this woman in her flowing, flowery dress, particularly grateful for the look of curiosity she focuses on him, as if he were simply another person. The café, despite the volume of the music, seems to him a thoroughly civilized place, with its flurries of cigarette smoke, its windowside table, to which a not overly garrulous waiter brings two glasses of cold white wine.

'You didn't find the talk this evening interesting then?' she asks him, after they have both taken a sip.

'It's not that. I've heard it before. In New York,' Robert coughs.

'A different version?'

'Not really. That's why I left.' He doesn't know quite why he stops himself explaining that Yvonne is his wife. 'And you?'

She shrugs, makes a comical face. 'I was never very good at school. Wanking or any other kind.'

Robert chortles. Her turn of phrase charms him as much as the turn of her lips.

'Let's have a look at your impulse buying, then.' She takes the magazines from him and flicks the pages with open interest. Then she shakes her head in exaggerated desperation, 'No, they do nothing for me. I guess it's that tired old cliché. Women do it to prose, men to images. Is that true, do you think?'

Robert wants to say that he finds it far more arousing talking to her here in this little space which is somehow secret than doing it at all. The sudden intimacy of the conversation has given him an almost forgotten sense of pleasure. But banter is an art that has gone into hiding, buried by censorship. So he says nothing at all, simply looks at her.

'Masturbation interests you?' She fingers a button on her dress as she says this.

Robert finds that his neck has grown inexplicably hot. He clears his throat with difficulty. 'As a public phenomenon. Though personally, I find other people more interesting.'

'Tell me about the phenomenon,' she urges him on. There is something brazen about her, as fearlessly bright as the anemones in the squat jug on the table. He concentrates on the flowers.

'You know . . . It signals a fear. A fear of other people. Particularly men. Makes them superfluous. And all of us into little security-wired islands, sufficient unto ourselves, with our videos and our images and our walkmans, our dial-a-pizza and dial-a-fantasy.'

Robert feels like a traitor as he says this. It is a good thing this woman doesn't know Yvonne is his wife.

She laughs. He would like to hold the anemones to her throat to see if the velvety centres are as dark as her eyes.

'You're a moralist,' she says then.

'Hardly,' Robert shakes his head, meets her laugh. 'Back home we have a few too many of them. I'm a lawyer. Perhaps we have too many of those as well.'

'You're nostalgic then,' she challenges him, 'You blame the women's movement?'

Robert balks at this. 'It's not as simple as that,' he says. 'Women's Lib was necessary. And I'm not in the business of blame.'

He can see she wants him to go on, perhaps so that she can disagree with him, but he wants to change the subject. He wonders how old she is. Thirty perhaps, older than his eldest daughter at least.

'What's your name by the way?' he asks.

'Tracy O'Donnell.'

'I'm Robert Bates.'

Robert stretches his hand out to her and notices a smile tugging at her lips. He wonders if she is about to link his name to that word. The Irish are good at puns. It's just as well, for a variety of reasons, that Yvonne has always used her own name.

To preclude his possible embarrassment, Robert rushes in and says, 'You know, I remember dresses just like yours the first time round.'

'The mill of fashion is jet-propelled these days.' She laughs again, her eyes crinkling. Robert likes the fact that she laughs so much. It comes to him that you can't masturbate and laugh at the same time. Perhaps that is the problem. He almost says this to her, but changes his mind. Instead, he focuses on her dress again.

'The vulnerable look. Isn't that what it's called?'

She nods, 'But the first time round, the pundits say, we wore them to look girlishly naughty but nice. And this time round the vulnerability . . .'

'Tells everyone you're victims or potential victims,' he finishes for her.

'Got it in one. We must have read the same piece.'

'Why would you want to look like a victim?' Robert asks with real interest.

She pauses for a moment. 'Women are, aren't they? That's why we have all this do-it-yourself sex,' she grins, then adds more seriously, 'Solidarity too, maybe. With the abused.'

Robert feels his smile growing tight. He knows about abuse from his practice. There is real abuse, which is horrible. And there is the desire to have someone named as an abuser, which brings its own red terror.

'Solidarity in reminding us men that we're beasts,' he says.

'Woman-eating beasts.' She is laughing at him.

But he wants her to understand. So he plunges in. 'What I

mean is that I don't see why women should want to get their sense of belonging from proclaiming themselves victims. After all, being victims gets you nowhere. All it does is allow you to point an accusing finger, turn all men into something they aren't. All.' Robert stumbles, realizes he has lost his way, has been portentous. He finishes a little lamely, 'Victim's logic. A vicious circle of vengeance. No people. Just categories. It becomes contagious.'

'Sad, isn't it.' She meets his eyes.

For a moment they are quiet, then she is all laughter again. 'You know, I think you might have a serious case of victim envy,' she says with an impish glance.

'I hope not.' Robert empties his glass. Her look reminds him of another, a playful world. He would like to wander in it. But she has gotten up.

'Got to dash. I'm late. You'll pay for the drinks.' She is all movement and he couldn't hold her back if he tried. But she stops, just as he is about to try to.

'Nice man, Robert Bates. Not a beast.'

The waiter brings Robert another glass of wine and he sips it slowly while he gazes at the anemones. By the time his wine is finished, he realizes Yvonne too will now be finished with the round of questions and interviews which inevitably follow these occasions. He makes his way across the darkened street and has to knock hard at the bookshop window to gain entrance.

Yvonne is leaning a little wearily against the platform table when he reaches the top of the stairs. She gestures him to her side, rests her fingers on his shoulder.

'Meet my husband, Robert Bates.'

'I'd recognize him anywhere. From the pictures.'

The woman from the café stretches her hand out to Robert. Squeezes it as he flushes.

'Ms O'Donnell is . . .'

'One of those *beastly* journalists,' Tracey O'Donnell finishes for Yvonne. She passes a copy of *Secret Pleasures* to her. 'You will sign this for me, won't you?'

While Yvonne signs, Tracey gives Robert a wink of flagrant conspiracy.

And despite the fact that he feels a little stunned, a little cheated and thinks he may be cited in the papers the next day as a porn monger, Robert has an unusual sense of elation.

Secret pleasures, he thinks. Yes, now he remembers them.

small death
in venice

sean o caoimh

They call it the small death but this, he thinks, is a long drawn-out agony.

He lies there, the grand horizontal, and she rides him hell for leather. He tries to stay hard and it obliges, taking its own pleasure. He watches it going in and coming out, a thing apart, working away, shining and flushed with pride. Remote as it is he wills it to pulsate, to twitch, to throb.

She says – You're marvellous, the best lover I've ever had.

He thinks – That's something. Score out of ten? The latest ten?

Outside the barges hit the pilings of San Trovaso. Rumble of diesels, shouts, hooting of vaporetti on the Grand Canal. In the Galleria dell'Accademia next door the cast out lady in Giorgione's *Tempest* sits naked under the town called Paradise.

Inside Room 12 of the Pensione Accademia she sits on his erection and heaves up and down and undulates like a turbulent sea. He lies there unmoved.

She says – I love it.

He looks up at her. Her face is contorted by her intense concentration. It's red and blotchy and sweat streaks her forehead. Eyes bloodshot, the whites veined in pink. She has the grim, tight-faced determination of a pained jogger or a cyclist leaning into a steep hill. She holds her breasts in her hands and throws her head back in military jerks in time with her hips.

He fills her. He matches her spasms with his convulsions. It's remote, detached, with a life of its own, but obedient to the cause.

He thinks – Now I'm just a cocksman. No lover no more.

She says – I want you to come.

He thinks – I'm saving it for Christmas.

He's irreverent, almost indifferent.

It wasn't always like this.

The meeting on the mountain at Verbier. The exchange of looks. The instant knowing. The trembling. In the village next day – Come to Venice. – Yes. Later that evening, the Visitation. His room filled with her fragrance, his bed with her lace, her skin, her delectable wetness. Her long hair brushing his cock. – It's beautiful. Is it mine? – Forever. What a laugh.

The small death and the resurrection. Again and again.

She says – I can't come any more. And comes again.

He's hooked. In deep, in love with her body, erotic love that's like drowning.

The narcosis of the cunt.

His desire: to be better than the rest.

A week later in Venice. Looking at the Veronese in the Palazzo Ducale. Europa abducted by the Bull. Her lips parted, her face in ecstasy, a wayward breast, abandonment. And the first shock.

He says – I'm like a bull when you make love with me.

She says – I fuck. I don't make love.

But she smiles and squeezes his bulging trousers.

In Room 12, disarray. She light and airy like an *île flottante*, her skin tasting as cool and fresh as the first salmon of the season and the first green peas. Him addicted. Lust into love and no protection. Compulsive touching. She holding his hard under the Titian in the Frari. His fingers inside her going up the steps in San Rocco.

Then, the illusion. The re-living of the moments, endowed with romantic love, profane yet sacred. The manic lift every time. The letters. The midnight calls: I miss you. And more. Each word remembered and inflated. The rerouting of life around her. The fitness of it; the certainty. The almost religiosity of it. Yes, the grand illusion.

Now she's alone, masturbating herself on him. And he's away in the Palazzo Labia coming off on the Tiepolos.

She says – I'm coming.

He thinks – Great. Best out of three?

He looks at her lumpy stomach. The sucked-in diaphragm, the tensed-up muscles running like a mountain range from rib-cage to pubis. A flat-topped ridge criss-crossed with deep ravines. The folded-up layers of flesh lined like the neck of an old sea turtle. Or a concertina. Everything in motion, sinews stretched, thighs lifting and falling like the connecting rod of a ship's reciprocating engine. And down there the beauty mark just above the crease of the V.

She says – I love it.

She leans over to watch herself as she pumps away, her hair mercifully hiding her face: she can't see his apartness, the falsity of his act. Now she reaches up, throws her head back, her mouth open, beginning to sound. She drops a hand and grabs his. She rubs it against her mons, her fingers touching his slippery cock.

She says – I want to kiss it.

She falls off and turns and kneels, *soixante-neuf*, and takes him in her mouth and offers him her sex. He extends a tentative tongue. He has lost the taste.

He remembers. The dunes. The golden sand in her golden hair. The taste of salt, of honey, of delicious cunt.

He thinks – How I loved her. Was there always hate underlying the love? It's too sophisticated for a bog Irishman with his prick still in the confessional.

She's on her way now. Eating him like a ripe mango. Her nether region vibrating in synch with her mouth and tongue. She holds nothing back. Always over the top. Gluttony in all orifices.

The small death. How did it expire?

With humiliation.

It keeps coming back. When she turned up with the finger bruises inside her thighs. Up by the slit. Black and blue from violent fucking. From learning to dive, she said, not caring that it was an obvious lie. Not important enough for a decent deception. Not caring.

She wants more than he can give. He had thought no one could give her more. He was naive. He asked her if she wanted two men, wanting her to be angry. She only laughed and said – The only aphrodisiac is variety, Baby. Lighten up.

By the pool. Raoul working on the fence. She beckoned. Then the three of them in the water, her holding them both. Raoul sitting on the side, her head between his legs and himself entering her from behind. Her laughing and him sick to death.

Upstairs. Her guiding him into the forbidden place while she lowered herself over Raoul. He could feel the intruder. The shit on the sheets.

She said – It's just a game. It doesn't count.

But it did. It does. Now she is there, all by herself. She raises her head, squeezes his prick hard, locks his head into her cunt, floods his face.

She cries – Oh, God! Oh, darling!

He thinks – Oh, balls. Change the record.

She lies on top of him and tries to eat his mouth. She tastes of cunty ashes. He tries to turn away. She pulls his head back. She's angry.

She says – You don't love me any longer.

He thinks of the old joke – Loves you? Of course I loves you. I fucks you, don't I?

He says – Let's go to the island of San Michele. With the mist and the cypresses.

She says – Yes, let's. It sounds sexy.

He wishes he could get a funeral gondola, all black and gilt, with four oarsmen and angels with wings spread on the stem and the stern, a black canopy with tassels, and cushions where the coffin lies.

The taxi-boat arrives at the ornate gate of the cemetery of San Michele. It's twilight. Long shadows, black water, smell of mud and putrescence. The lights of Murano filtered through the mist. Rose walls and sinister cypresses. They step ashore. He tells the man to wait. The man says it's closing soon. To hurry.

She says – It looks like a graveyard.

He says – Yes. A burial ground. L'Ile des Morts. It was once a prison.

She says – It is sexy.

He says – All the best people come here. Stravinsky. Diaghilev. Ezra Pound.

She asks – Who was he?

He says – A mad poet. We have to pay our respects.

They go to Ezra Pound's grave. It has a white stone and a white urn filled with fresh flowers. He stands. He turns to her. He lowers his hand. He unzips himself. He pushes her head down, not gently. She squats. She extracts his penis. It's hard.

She sucks him, he helps her by pulling it next to her mouth. His hand hits her teeth. Now she is excited. It's a new experiment. It's the kind of bizarre situation she likes.

He pushes her away and ejaculates over the grave.

She cries – Why did you do that?

He says – A benediction. He wrote about you: 'Your mind and you are our Sargasso Sea.'

She says – What does it mean?

He says – Weeds, darling, we're mired in weeds. Putrid, rotten, all passion spent.

He turns and walks away.

Small death in Venice.

Dead and buried.

R.I.P.

do you love me

marge piercy

Oily night pads in. The city reeks. It is hot in the room under the eaves of the townhouse, where they pitch in bed. To her, Edmund feels all spines. He penetrates her like a question and she responds with her hips nervously, shallowly.

'I don't know if I love you.' Edmund, whom nobody calls Ed, is sitting on the bed's edge, thinner than ever.

She shivers with sweat. 'Should I leave? Go back to New York?'

'Of course not.' Politely. 'Don't be melodramatic.'

'It's worse since we started sleeping together.'

'Worse?' He shoots to his feet, reaching for his briefs. 'What's worse? It's enough to make anyone nervous, tiptoeing around my parents' house.'

'Why do we stay here then? Let's go someplace else.'

'You said you liked them.'

'I do. Especially your father. He's a dear.'

He winces, misbuttoning his shirt. Waits for her to help him. In his angular face the grey eyes are set wide. They look past her, anticipating his flight down to the second floor.

Tossing on the cot after he has left, she hears dry voices, the ticking of glib excuses of the men who have borrowed and used her. Her fingers scrape the sheets. She is twenty-two and he is twenty-eight, an instructor who was her section man in philosophy, but she is his instructor in bed. She shares herself with him as a winning argument. But he takes her gingerly, and afterward, it is as if sex were something he had stepped in.

At school she had gone out with Edmund from time to time that last winter and spring, evenings he had taken more seriously than she had. People said she was pretty; she danced well; there were always men. She had been astonished when he proposed she spend the summer with him in his parents' home. He said they would learn a great deal about each other without being committed to anything, that she would like Boston and find their home comfortable. He was thinking about marriage: that amazed her. Therefore she did not say No, but Maybe. She took him home with her by way of testing, but learned little except that he settled easily into a placid boredom.

After her last finals she went off to New York, hitchhiking with her one suitcase. Her photographer boyfriend turned out to have a moneyed girlfriend he was living with. She stayed with friends, then other friends, sleeping on lumpy couches. She had imagined being an editor, making the delicate literary decisions she had been taught in school, but she was asked if she could type. She found a job so boring she would sometimes think she would die at her computer terminal in the long mornings and longer afternoons. They started to talk at her about dressing differently. She called Edmund in Boston.

Now the house encloses her, like an elbow. The house is as busy with a hundred concealed pursuits and escapes as a forest. His father talks to his mother; his mother talks to the black maid. She and the mother give each other little electric shocks. The father is okay – scotch-and-water, the Maine woods in hunting season, the local *Globe* and the New York *Times*, and a blown wistfulness in his thick face. The mother is tall and dry. She seems to move with the sound of tissue paper.

Coming into Edmund's territory, she finds that whether

they are to marry, whether he wants to, grows every day bigger and bigger. She rests in his hands like something inert.

Edmund lies in his ivory bedroom. He turns his cheek against his special firm pillow, drifting through his melancholy love for his married cousin Isabel – roses in waxy green paper, Limoges china. Soothing as his mother's hands in childhood fevers.

He feels her in her attic room pressing down on his head. Why did he bring her here? Often he cannot remember. Sometimes she resembles his dreams of the girl who will belong to him, but sometimes she grates. He is amused to think she was born in a Western where names are jokes, the town of Dogleg Bend where dust shimmies in the streets under a sky of mercury.

Once he went there with her, just before finals. Her waitress mother, fat and messy, greeted her without surprise. Her younger sister seized her and they remained closeted for hours. She spoke to no one on the streets. She took him around a maze of overgrown fields and swaybacked houses, playing guide as if there were anything to be seen: that's where we lived the year I was ten. That's where my sister Jeannie and I used to fish on the sandbar. There's where the Massey boys caught me when I was coming from the diner, and when I yelled, they jumped up and down on my stomach. That's where I saw a wounded goose, in fall when they come over.

He has brought her to his family as a welltrained retriever will bring something puzzling to lay at his man's feet and wait, expectant. Is it good? Do we eat it?

By breakfast-time the heat has begun to rise, seeping into the shuttered windows. Her face, cool from sleep, across the English marmalade and muffins and yesterday's flowers, seems young again, closed into itself. He wants to touch her.

His hearty father makes a joke about their wan morning

faces. His mother suggests with buttery kindness that the girl's dress is somewhat short for the street. All eyes pluck at the seams of bright (too bright?) cotton. Do they know? Their hopeful politeness enwraps him. Yes, they would be glad to spread her on that maid's cot, to serve her up to insure that he is whole and healthy. His mother has always read books on mind-repairing. 'Son, I want you to feel free to bring your friends home.' 'Remember you have nothing to be shy about.' 'I've asked Nancy Bateman – you know the Batemans' adorable younger daugher? – to dinner Friday . . .'

He says, 'Mother, Father, we're going to the cottage for a week. It's too hot here. It's unbearable.'

Her eyes leap from their private shade, but she only takes more jam and teases his father. He knows, in deep thankfulness, that she is pleased and will reward him with an easy day. She will take his wrist in a hard grip and pull him off to play tourists in his own city. All day she will ask nothing. All day she will turn them into magic children from a story. He wants to push away from the table and hurry out with her.

Coming back from the crossroads store with groceries, she looks at him beside her. She cannot imagine marriage. But she knows it is what makes a woman real, weights her to a name and place. That safe feeling she would seek walking in the old cemetery: names and dates neatly grouped in families, even the little babies accounted for. She wanted to get away as long as she can remember. But being a secretary is no better than being a waitress, except that her back and feet hurt less and her eyes hurt more.

He says, 'I thought you'd be more struck by the townhouse. We're proud of the wood panelling and the staircase. It dates from 1830.'

But all houses impress her. All other dogs have equally big bones. Walking beside him she catches her breath as they come over a hill out of the scrub oak and the ocean yawns ahead. She is surprised again how tall it is, how much sky it uses up. That blue yawn is her future. She will drown.

This cottage squats on the last dune, facing the sea. She puts down the groceries and sits at the white sea-blistered table. She sits still with concentration. On the table are shells and pebbles she has been collecting.

She says without inflection, 'I packed my suitcase.'

'I saw you. Why? How can you leave?'

'There's a bus that stops on the highway at four ten, the woman at the crossroads store told me.'

'Why? Where do you want to go? You quit your job.'

She lays out the pebbles in circles. 'You don't want me to stay, enough.'

He sees himself returning to the city without her. The air will prickle with questions. Suppose after she leaves, he changes his mind and realizes he wants her? 'Where will you go?' Her flimsy canvas suitcase stands at the door.

She picks sand from the ribs of a scallop shell. 'New York? Maybe I'll go West.'

Choosing a place so idly makes him dizzy. He sees her blown off like a grasshopper. People cannot just disappear. 'By yourself?'

His tedious jealousy of tedious young men. She smiles. Her heart is chipping at her ribs. The road comes over the last dune fitted to its curved flank in a question mark. She does not dare turn from him to go inside and look at the clock. Will she really have to go? Will she have to get on that dirty bus and use up her last few dollars on a cheap motel? She concentrates on his bent head: want me! Want me, damn you. She is not sure how much money she has in her purse and wishes she had counted it in the bathroom.

He is staring at his knuckles, big for the thinness of his hands and bone-colored with clenching. 'Do you love me?'

She turns her head. Her gaze strikes into his with a clinking, the stirring of a brittle windchime. He is thinking about girls, the difficulty, the approaching, his shyness, the awkward phone calls with silences that open under him like crevasses in a glacier. She is wondering what she is supposed to say. 'What do you care?'

'I have to know.'

His long milky face, pleading laugh, set of mismatched bones. He is gentle. If he does not touch her with passion, neither does he hurt her. That is very important, not to be hurt. 'Of course I love you.'

'Do you?' Once again he ducks to stare at his knuckles.

She must risk breaking the tension. She goes to read the clock.

'What time is it?' he calls.

She comes back to answer. 'Five to four. I hope I haven't forgotten anything.'

A strand of hair in the wash basin? Steel hands press on his shoulders: decide, decide. His father's voice, rising with the effort to contain his temper. 'Squeeze the trigger, Edmund, squeeze it. Come on, it won't wait for you all day. Do it!' The rabbit bolted into the tall grass. In his relief he shot. His father strode away. Be a man, be a man. Pressure of steel hands.

He has always been fastidious not to give pain. 'Let's walk down to the water.'

She shakes her head. 'Not enough time. I can't miss the bus accidentally, don't you see?' In New York it will be hot. She will call somebody. She will sleep on a couch, and the next day again she will go around to the temp agencies wearing pantyhose in the heat. Men will pester her on the street, Men will buy her supper and expect to lay her as payment. 'I can't sit here any longer waiting for you to decide if you love me – can I?' She claps the sand from her palms, hating herself for having listened to his quiet voice, for having given herself into his hands like a bag of laundry.

He cradles his head, elbowing aside the shells and pebbles. They move him, the sort of treasures a child might hoard. He feels wrong, not sure why. He hates the carelessness of men like his father, men in the fraternity of his college years whose act of power is to give pain. He does not know what he wants, only that everything is going away. She is about to walk off with that flimsy suitcase and leave him tangled here.

She reads his face – sullen, puzzled. He will let her go. Her skin crawls. One more defeat. 'Well, want to walk me to the crossroads? It's time.'

But he does not rise. 'Stay.'

Hope scalds her. She wants, wants so badly that surely she must win. 'Why let it drag on?'

'You know it's hard for me to figure out what I feel sometimes. I'm slow to react. I can't just decide like that.'

'You can tell if you love me. You could tell you wanted me here for the summer, before.'

He is afraid, but of what? Her leaving? 'But I do love you!' He breaks from his chair, snatches the suitcase from her. 'I do love you. I want us to stay together.' The words slam like a door he is finally through. He feels weak with relief. He has done the right thing. He too will have a wife. He will have a wife and children with his name.

'Then I'll stay.' She stands quite still. That blue future gathers itself in a wave and goes crashing over her. I've won! she tells herself. Now I'll be safe. Now I'll belong. And I'll be ever so good to him. I'll never take another bus. I'll never sleep on somebody else's couch again.

But her spine is water and her hands curl up remembering that vertical house, his parents with their expectant eyes, his ivory bedroom with its air of sickroom. His thin arms fold around her in a tight but formal embrace like an up-ended box.

the pink shoes

christopher hope

On weekdays Alma would come home from work and emphatically spread herself so that she deeply filled the basket-weave chair, beneath the photograph of Leopold Stokowski conducting an unknown orchestra in some distant black-and-white year. The orchestra stared up dimly at the conductor. The leader of the orchestra, a fat man, had settled on the edge of his violin a white handkerchief upon which he rested his chin.

Roger had met Alma at a party in Camden. Women seemed quite interested when he told them about his job.

'I make people semi-famous for three minutes.'

He had heard these women wondering aloud. Had they heard correctly? Roger weighed their hurtful surprise against known advantage. Among the would-be semi-famous, some ended up on his futon.

Alma hadn't asked him anything. She told him that she was a hunter-gatherer. Only when he heard her talking about the metaphysics of washing detergents did he realize she must be in advertising. She was there with a man called Valentine, a weightlifter, who wore a black body stocking and a red bandanna. His pectorals rippled with each sip of mineral water. It made Roger queasy. Though why this display of male musculature should so offend him he could not explain. Except to say to himself that there seemed too much of it.

As he was leaving Alma stopped him in the hallway.

'Someone said you don't drive.'

Roger said he'd never got round to it, somehow. Alma drove him home in her Japanese sportscar, its dashboard bathed in pinky/orange light. She spent the night on his futon and never said a word about Valentine the body-builder.

He remembered how generous Alma seemed to be that night. How she had been simply everywhere he reached.

Alma moved in one wet March morning, carrying a tapestry hold-all displaying the joys of mediaeval hunting in a French forest. Highly-strung royal hunting dogs pursued rabbits with eyes the size of saucers. Alma also carried two plastic bin liners full of shoes. Outside in the street stood a rented van. It took them three hours to transfer all her stuff into the flat.

Alma's mother presented them with a set of Walt Disney cartoon cells of Snow White and the Seven Dwarfs and a flock of wooden parakeets, from the jungles of Peru. The birds flashed emerald and pink, swinging from perches in the uncertain English light. This was how the hunted trout must see the feathered lure, Roger decided later. Alma's mother was an interior designer and this made it impossible to object to her profligate love of painted birds.

Alma's mother brought her lover along when presenting gifts. Florian was ginger-haired and very excitable, though he said little. When he became excitable, he wept. He collected women's rubber bathing caps. His collection stretched from plain white hoods, worn by women and Australian life-guards in the twenties and thirties, to the sprigged and petalled headgear in pastel colours more popular in the sixties.

What Florian saw in the bathing caps Roger never understood but it seemed to him decidedly odd. The women declared that Florian's fetish was rather 'sweet'. Florian brought a selection of swimming bonnets to Roger's flat from time to time, and fiddled silently with the chin straps. Or plunged his fist into their rubbery cranial interiors. The protesting squeak of the violated space set Roger's teeth on edge.

People struggled to see Roger and Alma as a couple. 'Roger and Alma?' They would shake their heads, bewildered. Roger, short and dark, pulling slightly at his rather protuberant lower lip. Tall, blonde Alma introduced him with a chopping motion of her sharp right hand. 'Rog. You know Rog.'

People did not know him. When they heard he produced a television programme lasting three minutes, devoted to allowing people to speak their minds on any subject of their choice, they looked sceptical. 'Sounding Off' was a forthright programme and Roger did not look like a forthright man. Alma's friends tended to put him to work. They said, 'Can we leave the drinks to you, Rog?'

Yes, the leader of the orchestra resting his chin in the white handkerchief reminded Roger of a suckling pig, its head on a platter.

Alma pointed out, in her crisp way, that everything seemed to remind Roger of the farmyard.

Did she mean barnyard?

Alma shot straight back: 'What's the bloody difference?'

There was, at least in his mind, quite a difference. There were farmyards and there were barnyards. The latter were full of roosters on dung heaps and cocks and hens, cows being led to bulls and stallions serving mares. And, at the back of his mind, his mother years ago, upon finding a tin of contraceptives in his sock drawer, tapping the golden tin with her forefinger and saying: 'I hope it's never said of you that you desired the behaviour of the barnyard.'

That was exactly what he wanted. The behaviour of the barnyard. He wanted it in great muddy chunks: dunghill, roosters, stallions and all. Above all he wanted it with Alma.

When she lay back in the basket-weave chair beneath the photograph of Stokowski. When she reached up and played with the six brightly painted wooden parakeets swinging beneath the overhead lamp. When she kicked off her pink shoes and sent them sailing heaven knew where, and pointed her toes at the ceiling. When she accepted the money he'd given her, an unexpectedly large sum returned to him by the Inland Revenue, saying calmly that this was something she felt he owed her. When she showed the kind of burliness that knocked people over if they stood in her way, people who thought because she was slender and blonde she couldn't knock people over, until they saw her from the back striding away into the distance on her surprisingly long legs.

But most especially when she lifted her legs as she did now in the lamplight. Perfectly circular hollows between ankle and heel. Roger ached to wet the tip of his forefinger and slowly polish the divine hollows of Alma's ankles. Spit would do, or bath water. Oil of Evening Primrose. Steam. Soap. But all these things required time, leisure, space.

There was less and less space in their Bayswater flat. Alma had a way of spreading herself. The pink parakeets from Peru. Three dozen Victorian perfume bottles, ribbed with stippled silver. Three vintage barometers, four Halogen lamps, two VCRs. The larger of the two, said Alma, was 'state of the art'. It stood on the small cane table opposite their bed: black, bold, shapely, impossibly expensive. This, thought Roger, is how the Israelites must have felt when they worshipped the Golden Calf. And he bumped his knees in the narrow channel Alma had constructed between the wall and their bed.

Her bed, really. She had locked his futon in the cupboard. She had found the four-poster in a Chelsea loft one day while looking for old maps in the home of a friend of her mother. Alma loved maps. Those in their bedroom showed the reefs off the Shetlands.

'I'm ecumenical when it comes to maps!'

And she would lick her finger and stroke the glass as if she could feel the mountains, rivers and ridgy contours, like the armoured plates of some primitive sea monster, lying fathoms deep in the waters off the Shetlands.

In the evening Roger usually took up a defensive position in the hooded porter's chair in the corner, placed exactly between the window and the bookcase from where he watched Alma fill the chair and kick her pink shoes into the air, pointing her toes at the ceiling.

He had bought the pink shoes from the Azerbaijani boutique in the Fulham Road. An original creation, they had cost him a small fortune. With their stubby heels and projectile toes, he knew Alma would like them. Their pink was as much a matter of texture as shade. A hue somewhere delicately between raw veal and exposed human flesh. A pink, though he did not say so, the colour of Alma's tongue. A pink he could taste, veined with a ruddier flush towards toes and heels.

Alma liked to sleep naked, turned on her side, her face towards the luminous glow of the radio clock, casting a pink gleam on her hair. Surrounding Alma was what she called her 'air-exclusion'. And what Roger secretly referred to as his 'no-fly zone'. Carefully not entering the no-fly zone beside him, Roger pictured himself as a sharp arrow cutting through the air. He lay back with his eyes closed, listening as Alma rhythmically drew in oxygen and gave out carbon dioxide with long and perfect exhalations.

Sometimes he had what amounted to an out-of-body experience. He floated above himself and saw thin Roger below in the bed, well outside her air exclusion. Roger 'out of the body' would lean down and draw a line around the body of Roger 'in-the-bed', the sort of silhouette police drew in chalk at the site of murders and road accidents, to indicate where the body had been, pale evidence of someone who had been there.

Alma had a talent for taking over, a fluid imperialism. Most people had some capacity to flow. Even Florian got his fist into the cranial hollows of rubber swimming helmets. But Roger got nowhere. He was increasingly stuck. A dry stick. A bone on a deserted beach.

Night after night he lay in the big four-poster and grew slighter. He reduced his shirts, on their single shelf, from eight to four. He soon owned only two pairs of shoes. He gave his third jacket to an Oxfam Shop. And he hung his remaining jackets on a single hanger. Standing on Alma's bathroom scales he saw he had lost weight. He looked in the bathroom mirror, cleared the steam to check the fact and conceded that he was also losing hair. Each week was a narrow corridor at the end of which stood a closed door. To open that door, the slightest crack would do, was Roger's obsession, and to slip beneath it like a doorstop before it closed again.

Roger aimed the arrow of himself towards Saturday night. An hour before Alma awoke on Saturday morning he had set the table for breakfast. Later her bath, firstly warming her huge fluffy pink towel upon the heated rail, adding just enough bath foam to cover her body as she slipped beneath the water with a sigh and lifted her feet onto the edge of the bath. And then, pretending to brush his teeth while watching her in the steamy mirror. If things were destined to go well, he would hear her say, 'take your toothbrush out of your mouth, Rog.'

He might then coat the tip of his finger with shampoo and slowly polish the circles below her ankles while Alma hummed a bit from *Tosca*. Sometimes he forgot to take his toothbrush out of his mouth.

On Saturday nights in his indecent haste how often Roger banged his knees in the narrow channel between the wall and the bed as Alma reclined on the soft white hills of her three pillows.

'I really don't see it,' Alma said. 'I know lots of women do. But, frankly, I don't.'

'Tomorrow is Sunday,' Roger babbled. 'You can sleep in.'

But she didn't see it.

One evening Alma sent her pink shoes in a wide arc to land with a soft thump on the rug. She pointed her toes at the ceiling and, as if at a signal, the doorbell rang and there in the hall stood Valentine, the weightlifter, his sportsbag slung around his broad shoulders. Alma said, 'Hello stranger. You're in the pink.'

Valentine, it seemed, was working out at the gym during the day. He was a night club bouncer in the evenings. He wore a purple singlet and his muscles leapt when he sipped his mineral water. What was in his sportsbag, Alma wanted to know.

Roger picked up the copy of Virgil and began reading about the Fall of Troy. Valentine went into the bedroom and came out wearing a tiny triangular patch of black and yellow cloth, held up by shoelaces. Alma nodded approvingly:

'What's the good of a posing pouch if you don't pose?'

Valentine got on the table and Alma fetched a bottle of baby oil from the bathroom. The muscles of Valentine's calf inflated wildly as she rubbed. Dark blue veins branched and throbbed. No one paid any attention when Roger left the flat. His going was too slight to be noticed.

He arrived home after midnight. He had not gone more than a few steps in the darkness when he tripped and fell heavily. He lay there for a few moments, aware of the faint lingering smell of baby oil, before getting painfully to his feet and finding the light switch. Alma's pink shoes lay where Alma had kicked them.

'Lethal,' said Roger.

Alma was sleeping soundly, breathing out carbon dioxide.

Roger shook her awake and handed her the tapestry hold-all with the fleeing hares and the thin, pursuing hounds.

'You gave me those shoes,' she said accusingly.

It took her a minute to rub sleep from her eyes. Then she dressed. At the door she said, 'You're doing yourself a bad turn, Roger.'

'Your shoes are in the bag.'

He sat up all night in the porter's chair, reading about the Fall of Troy. At eight in the morning, a moving van arrived. It took a couple of men several hours to carry Alma's stuff from the flat. This was the sort of thing that went on when a government fell and the Prime Minister had to leave the official residence.

The flat was quiet, huge, empty. Roger fetched his futon from the cupboard and threw it on the floor. Lying on his bed a yellow triangle caught his eye. Valentine's posing pouch. Using Virgil and a copy of *A Shropshire Lad* to lift it from its hiding place under the cupboard, Roger carried the article to the kitchen, pressed tightly between two good books, intending to drop it in the rubbish bin. But as he passed the bathroom he got lost in all the space Alma had left behind. In the bathroom mirror stood a thin man, watching him. Between his paper paws he held the scrap of yellow cotton, its drawstring hung down like the tail of a mouse in the jaws of a barnyardcat, like something he had caught and killed.

sweet
nothing

jill neville

'Why do you surround yourself with second-rate people?'

'I wonder what they think about *you*?' I throw a cushion at him (the one my fiend of a husband bought in Bali), which he fails to catch. The man can't even catch a cushion. There he sits, his usual ungainly self, having spent the evening running down all my friends; hauling himself up to his feet from time to time to thump his chest and haunches until he locates one of those little bottles of Scotch he keeps stuffed in various pockets, never offering anyone else a drop. Whenever he moves there's a faint clinking sound.

On his bitter face the eczema that dried and raddled his skin long ago has flared up again. Why won't he leave? The others have all toddled off. They know I have to get up early to feed the baby.

After the Fiend I had a tentative affair or two; the first with a jazz musician who wore purple shoes. In our hot, moist bed we could have cultivated a new breed of tropical fruit; but his long silences were not eloquent. I heard him make only one remark that had not been pumped out of him and he spoke it in an undertaker's voice: 'I come from Gravesend. And it really is the grave's end.' It seemed to explain the purple shoes and the inarticulacy. The next contender was an architect perpetually incensed by all irrationally designed space, including delightful old vicarages with upstairs landings that led nowhere. He was always trying to persuade me to leave this huge, cheap, sombre basement with its dumb-waiter in the hall and move in with him, to his more rational premises. But like the vicarage landings it all led nowhere.

Almost every evening friends and friends of friends drop around; some of them desultory suitors, not sure about taking on someone else's baby. I serve coffee, keeping them at bay, like Penelope, but without any Odysseus in the offing. This evening Oliver Shankforth delivered a furious monologue on the corruption of the poetry Mafia in London. Rival poets were more vicious than hit-men and should be prevented from entering civilized communities.

'I suppose that scribbler Shankforth is in love with you too.' Stan thumps the Fiend's cushion as if he has something against it.

'I've told you before – he drops in when he's at a loose end because he lives next door. His latest girlfriend drives a Jaguar, but she doesn't like the colour. So she leaves it unlocked in dark alleys hoping someone will steal the thing – then Daddy will buy her a prettier one.'

Stan cackles. 'Well, at least he isn't a bore like your other hangers-on.'

You old shrivel-shanked poisonous bastard, get out of my hair and out of my life. I yawn dramatically.

He settles deeper into the chair and surveys me thoughtfully. 'I've stayed behind because I've got something very special to ask of you. I've been thinking about this for some time and I'm quite, quite serious.' He's gone absolutely still; a pre-pounce stillness. 'I'm offering you two thousand pounds in cash – if you go to bed with me for one night.' He gives me one of those rare naked looks people keep in store for emergencies.

My laughter lasts for some time. I am twenty-three and still buoyant despite the Fiend; despite debts. Stan is just being his usual preposterous self.

The first time someone brought him to my place he confessed that when he was young his ambition was to see naked women, 'lots and lots of naked women.' That meant he would have to become either a doctor or a painter, but Medicine involved too much hard work, so he chose the easier option. Later he took me off to that basement café in Queensway: The Artist's Palette, where *au pair* girls make a few extra bob posing naked for coffee-drinking lechers who have to pretend to be bona fide painters. Uneasily they sport black berets or carry easels, but read the sports news on the sly when they're not sliding their eyes over the nudes who sit displayed above them on a dais. Stan refused to wear a beret; simply pointed to his paint-spattered shoes. One amateur model had rolls of flesh on her belly and sat in a humiliated crouch. Stan insisted I notice the soft silvery light emanating from her skin. 'She's not used to being gazed at in public, so she's still got her secret light you see. But that other girl, her skin's got no aura at all. It's been looked to death.'

At his studio he offered to give me any painting of my choice. I was humbled then and thought I put too much emphasis on his eczema, his extreme age (he was about fifty), his clanking armour of little Scotch bottles. None of it counted because he could paint like this. I chose one of a seated woman, her hand under her chin contemplating the Artist. He grabbed it away from me violently and said he'd changed his mind. That made me gasp. But his bad behaviour always tickled me; from my safe distance.

'Two thousand pounds. Think about it.' His eyes are staring at me with that faraway yet concentrated beam. Those eyes belong in another face altogether, that of an artist before life crucified him; or a river god. But his lips twist in anticipation of my moral defeat. He enjoys endless proof of human frailty. He knows exactly how broke I am. He knows I lie awake at night worrying about pounds, shillings and pence.

'I've just received a summons to Marylebone Magistrates' Court for an unpaid bill of fifteen pounds.' I am collecting coffee mugs and ashtrays. He turns to follow my every move; his thin face with that permanently rankled look is daring me to prostitute myself. Two thousand pounds to go to bed with the old sod; to hold on to the side of the mattress and think of England – I'd sooner levitate.

I know very little about him except that he has been married a couple of times and each marriage is surrounded by a stench of scorched earth.

'Here, have a swig.' First time he has offered me a drink in his life and I need one. What a day. The baby banged her head on the fender. The landlord threatened to evict me. Oliver Shankforth was cold and cross when I told him I had written a sonnet about him. Stay out of the poetry racket was all he said. I accept one of Stan's little bottles and pour it into a tumbler. It's all right to drink now because I've stopped breast feeding.

'Two thousand pounds! I could paint my flat, buy clothes, pay debts, hire baby-sitters.' I am playing with him, giving him some of his own medicine. But he can tell by my tone of voice that it's out of the question. I am like that fat *au pair* girl at The Artist's Palette with the quivering light in her flesh. My flesh is still the mirror of my soul, darn it.

'Keep your claws off that Shankforth man. He's too snobbish for you. He'll marry some Sloane Square Samantha. And he'd never take on another man's baby. I would though.'

'Ha! Fine mess you've made of your marriages.' As he gives up hope about buying me his face is losing its rancour; I see sad sweetness there. Why is he always so strenuously awful? I suppose because he can get away with it. He sells his canvasses to the Tate. The critics drool.

'I like your hair back. You know it's the hope in your eyes that scares me. Don't you know the world is a pile of shit?

Hasn't anyone ever told you that a pessimist is an optimist with all the facts?'

Hope; I used to stare at her in the G.P. Watts painting up on the wall at home; blindfolded and bound, with the world beneath her sinking into the mire. She knows something will turn up; the cavalry, a change in fortune, divine interference, Mr Right.

'Do you often get obsessed with girls, Stanley?' The Scotch is rushing about my blood. And I have little resistance because I haven't drunk for so long; for one thing I can't afford it.

'I have only one obsession – work.' He staggers to his feet. 'Without obsession you don't achieve a thing. You just drift like pooh-sticks down the river until one fine day you look in the mirror and see a shrivelled ugly mug that reminds you of your grandad. And what have you achieved? *Sweet nothing.*'

'But, you're famous.'

He sits down again and his legs bounce up in the air revealing for a moment the flesh between his trousers and socks which seems to be covered in little scabs. He's so awkward, as if he's been incorrectly assembled. Was that his bones or his bottles clicking together?

'Perhaps a few oils; one or two sketches . . . have you eaten? You let that crowd slurp Nescafé but you never offer a sandwich. You starve us out.'

'I'll knock up something.' I feel guilty because I find him so sexually unattractive and I know just how much that hurts, because Oliver Shankforth finds me sexually unattractive. Oh yes.

'You have Egyptian shoulders.'

'Stop that.'

'Have some more of my lovely Johnny Walker. Keeps on keeping on.'

'I'll put on the spuds. Back in a minute.' In the kitchen I hum; the tap runs over icy fingers. Stan follows to fill up my drink; doesn't he know however drunk he gets me it's no use – I'll never agree to his proposition; and I'm not frightened of him, or threatened; he's so skinny I could fell him with one blow, poor old bugger. And his eczema! Hope it's not catching.

I slice open a cabbage; prick sausages and place them in the frying pan. I look up and see he's sketching me on the back of the summons to the Magistrates' Court.

'I want to fully comprehend your bone structure lady; you are so odd and so beautiful at the same time.'

'Flattered, I'm sure.' Stanley is standing a bit too close; and the hour is a bit too late for him to be here. His woman, Margie, the one who phones him from time to time, will phone him soon, sobbing and pleading, and he will be rude to her. Of course she will presume the worst. She turned up once when I was alone in the afternoon: a battered blonde, tousle-haired, red-eyed, dripping poison at me, asking me what my game was.

'I have no game.'

'You're after him. After his money.'

My indignant denials, my talk of friendship merely darkened her suspicions.

'Careful Stan, you'll get scalded.' Why am I cooking meat and two veg for this scarecrow at midnight? It's not my fault that he's in love with me. Let him roll like a coconut in the hold of the tossing ship.

'If we do it we'll have to do it with the lights off. All I ask is a little reciprocation.'

'Reciprocation?' It comes out like *reshiproshation*. I must stop drinking; must eat something.

We are half way through the meal when, predictably, the phone rings. Wearily I answer it. Wearily I hand him the receiver.

'You bore me,' he says, and hangs up.

'God you're mean. She loves you.'

'Listen Madam, I'm taking my offer back. You've cost me far too much already – a whole year of abject misery. It would be cheaper to sell my studio, buy a diamond from Cartier and throw it into the Thames.'

'Friendship, Stanley, is two pooh-sticks floating down the current side by side.'

'Sounds like a good marriage.'

'You'd be incapable of that. I pity your ex-wives and that woman Margie. Poor Margie.'

He puts his head back on the sofa and stretches out each arm in the crucified position. 'Do you know why I'm in the top league of British painters? They love me because I've got *vigour* and that's rare in British art. But I'll tell you a secret and if you go blabbing it about town I'll personally see to it that you are killed.'

'Don't tell me then.'

'I'm half-Jewish.'

'So?'

'If they knew I was Jewish they'd lose interest. They'd say – he's not a unique British painter after all, just some clever Jewboy.'

'It must be nice to have power . . . fame . . .'

'Nicer to have beauty.' He feels by entering me he would enter this beauty he sees in me. Now his eyes are the eyes of old-fashioned hopeless longing. So sad. So sweet. Suddenly I feel a cramp of pity.

I leap up and collect the plates. Neither of us ate much; we had left it too long. 'I'll make coffee.'

I'm in the kitchen now, scraping leftovers on to a piece of newspaper, waiting for the kettle to boil. I wrap uneaten food in the paper and bend down to stuff the bundle in the bin; can't afford no pedal bin; no pedal bin for the likes of little old me. I am swaying. I feel dizzy. I stagger. I drop the bundle on to the linoleum. I go down on my knees to clear up the mess. Then I stop and stare. Stanley is staring straight up at me. The same famished face. The same tunnelling eyes. The shrivelled lips. Not hiding behind masks of mockery. This is a portrait of the artist as himself. A very needy person. I stay crouched on the floor, swaying a little, head still spinning. Why has Stanley's photograph got into *The Sunday Times*? I push aside the cabbage and see that it is an Oxfam advertisement. I stare into the Oxfam face, into Stanley's Oxfam face, into his starving soul. I look at all the wasted food I'm throwing away. Why does it always have to be like this? I'm sick of the whole stupid, unfair world. Why can't we simply post our dinners straight into the mouths of the suffering millions?

I stand up. For once the hungry will be fed. There will be no middlemen, no bureaucrats to syphon off the goodies. It will go to the hungry – not to the Oliver Shankforths of this world who have their Carolines and Veronicas lining up in their daddies' shining cars. No, poor old Stanley with his eczema and his bile, he's the one who must receive my love. I will offer him the inimitable secret of my luminous sexuality. Poor old Stanley. Let us join bodies. Let us make love the night through. When the baby wakes I shall be tired, but no matter. This night is a night that is the night that is the night that is happening tonight.

I turn off the kettle. I float down the hall, winged with purpose. My maternal milk has boiled over to cover the universe. I pause at the threshold, and summon him. He is crouching miserably; sober, sad; *sad*, no matter how deeply he drinks of his elixir of death. He frowns at me. A line of poetry Oliver Shankforth once quoted comes into my mind:

> The frowning schoolgirl may
> Be dying to be asked to stay.

'*Stanley*.' He looks up at me.

I look up at her. She is standing at the door without holding any mugs of coffee. She has a curious gleam in her eyes. She is standing in a different way; what is it? Something has clarified; or obscured; what is it? She smiles. She is smiling a slow emphatic smile. Is it? The old heart lurches. I stand up. The wretched bottles clink. She is beckoning me. I am undefended against my own sense of wonder. I get up jerkily. My body moves in segments like an insect. God I'm repulsive. But I walk towards her, clinking faintly. She takes me by the hand. I put my clammy, eczemaed hand in her young warm grip. She leads me silently down the long basement corridor, pausing for a moment to listen at her baby's door, then onwards, past the dumb-waiter through the chaos of the tiny kitchen which smells of boiled cabbage (this woman wouldn't make a good third wife) and into her bedroom which has an uncurtained skylight. If she puts the light on she'll see me naked. She'll scream.

In this room I've never been allowed to enter before, dark except for the nightclub glow from the paraffin heater, a skirt slithers to the floor. The pupils of my eyes expand to absorb her body, back-lit in red, as she lifts one leg and places her foot on the bed and unpeels a black stocking. Suspenders un-click on pale thighs; elastic bounces back inside bunched petticoats. She bends lower, raising the arch of her foot, working the hose over her heel; one eye visible as she peers up at me and grins. 'Don't trip over the bucket, Stanley.' She's a Toulouse Lautrec; the naughty immortal whore undressing; louche as the ping of leaking rain in the old tin bucket.

I want the light on in order to see her in bed. But she must not see the monster soon to be on top of her. Perhaps there's just enough light washing through the ivy-encrusted skylight, hazy with the soft nibble of London rain. Because there's a moon of sorts.

I rip off my jacket, an awkward bottle-clinking business. I am standing wrestling with my sleeves, arms akimbo, a scarecrow in love. I struggle with my trousers, avoiding the bucket. 'You should complain to the landlord about that leaking roof.' My voice is trembling. 'You shouldn't let him exploit you.'

She is taking off her sweater. It is over her face. Only her neck is visible, the Egyptian shoulders, the long Modigliani waist. Her arms swing down. She throws the sweater into a corner, unleashes her breasts; two bouncing pears, and below them the dark triangle.

She rushes into bed like a child. I follow. One of my feet touches one of hers. She withdraws it as if shot. If only she'd massage my icy feet. Get the circulation going. Lick me all over, lick the unlicked cub. Redeem me. She is going too fast, to get it over with, like the washing-up.

If you could only desire me there would not be this banal tussle, this mess. You would stand in the middle of the room, my little nut tree with your silver nutmeg and your two golden pears and I, old Mr Bones, would go down on my bony knees. Perhaps, given time, you would dance for me in black underwear. And as I watch you I will grow attractive. Your beauty will transform this bad old beast.

I pull down the blankets. I want to see you, see you in a sexual trance. You have gone back centuries; a Titian goddess in your bower of falling stars and dirty sheets smelling vaguely of baby's bottles. I place a hand on your breast. You shiver as if you're in the North Pole, yet the paraffin fire is glowing in the corner. The female nipple is the barometer of pleasure. It cannot lie as the vagina can. Yours fail to respond. So I resort to a kiss. I give it the same determination I give a recalcitrant canvas. I press through mouth, teeth, tongue until I enter the ridged wetness of your interior; but there's too much tension in your spine. You are steeling yourself up for the ordeal like a virgin.

Perhaps the baby was an immaculate conception; or does Aphrodite renew her virginity after every erotic adventure? No. It's no good. You won't let yourself go. I lie back and stare up at the evil, grinning, voyeuristic moon.

You leap upon me like leaping into the chilly North Sea, your breasts dangle over my chest, but you weigh too heavily. What a whacking great wench you are after all, with a Rubenesque bum. You heave yourself up. You move lightly up and down my torso tickling me with your breasts, then start to toil away down there, toiling in the salt mines of your man's cock. I lie back, receiving it, plying my fingers in your spread-out hair. The trouble with waiting too long is you always make a hash of it first time. But now I lie back in gathering animal bliss as the rain goes ping-ping-ping in the bucket. Suddenly I must act. I turn you over and you're as light and starry as the delectable Cranach Eve.

Once I saw you scrubbing the baby's floor, back and forth, back and forth, the immemorial female rocking; scrubbing and fucking are somewhat similar movements. That's why gentlemen always want to screw their maids. When this is over I want you to walk about the room confident as Olympia while I lie back drinking, sketching, *sated*. I want to divine the golden-green in your skin, your tumbled hair, the fullness of your fruiting breasts, your unfathomable cheerfulness. I start to babble into your moist ear. 'I'm going to take out a Covenant on you. Five thousand pounds a year. It could come out of my Supertax.' I am spending, spending, I will give it to you. Give, give. Oh wondrous bitch. You're responding. You're moving with me. I've activated the primitive mechanism at last; something staggered out of the Ice Age; out of the six-million-year swamp. The smell of sea-slime and almonds. And your eyes as you look up at my dribbling, soon to ejaculate self are dreaming. Oh Muse of my Desire that knows no shame.

'Stanley. Please stop. I can't go through with this. I'm terribly sorry.'

I stall. A warthog over my prey. '*You bitch*'. The erection shrivels. The room shrivels. The poison returns to the poison-glands. You stare up at me, eyes blank as granite, a Henry Moore abstraction of Woman reduced to a hole; the poor forked female creature with monumental power. You're throwing me out even though your cunt was saying yes, even though your cunt, like a murderer's mongrel was being its cheerful compliant doggy self. Did you take me to bed out of pity? Out of charity? Was this a charity-fuck? Part of your moist maternity? You little girl from Nowheresville with your poorman's *soirées*, go fuck your way through the *Penguin Book of Modern Verse* because you ain't got no talent yourself. In a few years you'll bulge like a George Grosz tart.

On the bedside table there's a teething ring. Yes, you're already a used body, a potential old bag. With your capricious nature no wonder the Fiend fucked off. I'd be curious to meet him. We'd have something in common. Like two Nam Vets. I throw on my clothes and nearly trip over the bloody bucket while you go on whining. I'm sorry. Ping. I just couldn't. Ping. Forgive me. Ping. I was drunk. Ping. I jerk on my jacket and if a bottle falls and breaks let it. May she step on the shards in the morning. That noble face is a ploy of Nature's. She's like the rest of 'em. Except Margie. Margie looks like a plum pudding. But Margie has one great advantage: she wants me.

Stanley bangs the front door. Can Oliver Shankforth hear it? I cringe under twisted sheets. But I have to get up to see if the baby has woken, afraid of the unknown world boiling around her. She remains asleep, exhausted by having to breathe noisily through adenoids. She makes me weak with love and responsibility. I put on the kettle. I have lost a friend; nothing to celebrate; I could have tamed him into a friend. I take the tea back to bed. I should have gone through with it; continued to lie under piles of dead ashes – what was it they used to snigger in my ear at school? *Marry an old man and feel old age creeping over you.* Ah, the dankness of his flesh, the coldness of his spittle. But why couldn't I be generous? Why is desire so inflexible? It operates with Oliver Shankforth whom everyone in the world wants. It operated with the Fiend who was cruel and with Purple Shoes who was dumb-struck, but with the one who loves me, a tortured genius, desire has to sulk; sit in its den and suck its thumb and if forced out it throws a tantrum. I'm itchy now; Stan's eczema. Serves me right; my punishment for going against the great power of that bastard Eros. I will miss Stanley. We were Beauty and the Beast in reverse. I couldn't turn him into a Prince but he turned me into a goddess. And I will miss his audacity. I turn off the lamp and watch bits of grated moon peeking through ivy leaves. The rain has stopped nagging me now. The bucket is silent. Tomorrow I must empty it; empty it of today's mistake. I shall leave the paraffin heater on until it runs out; bask until dawn in its expensive glow; a comfort, like buying a hat when you've been fired. One day I will dream of Stanley; still guilty. But he will look down at me from dream-heaven with radiant affection because he will be dead then and understand everything.

The baby snorts in her sleep. The wind makes its quiet shushing around the battered London house and I can go to sleep now too, despite the itchiness.

christmas
present

victor headley

Scalding hot, the spray of water splashes on his foot. Swearing, Robin withdraws it quickly, fiddles with the knobs until he gets the temperature right. He steps in fully this time, lets the downpour soak him all over. At first he tries not to get his hair wet; with the freezing weather outside he's bound to catch a cold. But then he gives up on that. As the water beats down on the top of his skull, Robin tries to shake off the bad feeling. He knows only too well he shouldn't be here this morning but last night again he gave in to Lizzie. How many times now has he been in this shower, how many mornings feeling angry at himself for obeying his impulses? Robin scrubs himself furiously as if the soap could somehow wash away what he feels. Through the noise of the rushing water, Robin hears her voice calling out from behind the door. Frowning, he doesn't answer. He hears Lizzie enter the bathroom. She pulls open the shower curtain. Robin wipes away some soap from his face, opens his eyes and sees her standing there in a purple nightgown. She's got a cigarette in her hand. He says nothing, feels her gazing over him.

'Are you going?' Lizzie asks.

At times like this, Robin hates even the sound of her voice, the way she speaks. He throws her a cold stare from under the waterfall and pulls the plastic curtain shut. One full minute passes, smoke drifting lazily upwards to the ceiling. Then slowly the curtain slides open again. Lizzie is still standing on the same spot, but the gown has fallen crumpled at her feet, the cigarette has disappeared. Robin is about to say something, something not very nice, but before it happens, Lizzie takes one step forward and climbs into the shower. She spins around, water crashing down on her shoulders. It splashes on her chest, runs between her cream-coloured breasts. Robin has stopped washing now; in his mind a voice is saying 'get out!' He knows that voice, the same one that warns him every time he's about to surrender to his nature. And sure enough, this morning like all the other times before he hesitates. And like every other time, that hesitation, the few seconds after this inner voice has spoken, brings his downfall. The next thing he knows, Lizzie's long and slender fingers are caressing his chest, her long nails gently scratching his wet skin. There's still time to break it up ... Robin knows he ought to stop looking into the brown eyes now piercing into his. With her lips on his neck, his back touches the glass of the shower wall behind him. Then it's all over with his resistance. He hears himself saying, weakly, 'Stop ... I've got to go to college.' The words are lost as Lizzie presses on, working on him. He loses what little lucidity he's been hanging on to, she traps him, takes him over ...

Robin is doing his best to resolutely ignore Janet's questions and disparaging remarks. She's between the cooker and the fridge, to and fro, pausing by the table to glance at him before returning to her cuisine. That's the last thing Robin needs tonight; his sister is known for her ability to chat non-stop, especially when it comes to admonishing him. Robin knows the phone call from his course tutor got her started. If only he had made it to college today, he could have sorted out this whole thing! But no, he had to waste his time in Bexley and now, exhausted and disgruntled as he feels, he's got to put up with the incessant nagging of his older sister.

'You're not answering me?'

Robin looks up. Janet is standing there, a knife in one hand, an onion in the other, eyeing him suspiciously. He sighs.

'What was the question?'

'Oh, so you're not listening to me!'

The dinner he has only just touched has lost its appeal. Robin puts down the fork, gets up from the table.

'Look Janet, I have some things on my mind. I'll sort out everything, don't worry.'

Janet seems dubious about that. Shaking her head, she turns to the cooker and gets busy. Robin goes to the fridge, pours himself a glass of juice, feeling like he hasn't slept for days.

'We have a deal, I hope you remember that!'

Janet won't let go of the subject, not that easily. Robin knows that only too well. Every time she even thinks he's going off the track, she keeps mentioning it.

It was nice of her to take him in the previous year. At that time, after the blazing row with their parents, Robin wasn't sure where he would have gone. But he was determined not to stay at home one more day. The only thing Janet had demanded from him was that he'd attend college regularly and pass his grades. That was fair enough and Robin had done quite well, until two months ago. 'I remember and I'll stick to it, okay? Take it easy.'

It's best to leave the kitchen or Janet will go on and on. At 23, she's only five years older than him but to Robin she's sounding more and more like their mother already. He gets to his bedroom, crashes on the bed with relief. Tomorrow is Saturday, that means rest, all day. Robin almost falls asleep there and then but finds the energy to undress. This must be the first time he has ever gone to bed at 8 o'clock on a Friday evening. The light off, Robin dives into oblivion, not before a last fleeting vision of Lizzie's face flashes through his mind.

Life had been pretty much peaceful and predictable until the woman came into his life. The first time at college was fine, as was everything else. During the week, apart from the twice weekly training sessions at his kung fu club, Robin concentrated on his homework. He'd spent time with Danny, his long time partner, playing chess and listening to music but on the whole, leisure time was weekend. Generally the Friday evenings were reserved for Marlene. They'd go to the movies or just stay indoors. Sometimes a party on the Saturday night.

Marlene doesn't demand but since she goes to college outside London and stays by her aunt in the week, she rightly expects to see Robin for most of the weekend. They've been going out together since the previous summer and everything has been just nice between them. Until the end of the year that is.

The Christmas party at Janet's office is where it all began. Robin thought he'd go along with her and spend some time there, warming up for his own later ravings. He had a few drinks, met some of his sister's colleagues and was mingling in a convivial atmosphere when he first noticed her looking at him. She was having a conversation with some other people near the buffet but Robin could feel her eyes on him right across the room. He thought nothing of it until shortly after when he went for a refill.

'Hello, do you work here?'

Robin turned to his right and found himself staring into those same eyes that had been seeking his earlier. He was still holding the bottle of sparkling white wine. She smiled, motioning him to pour some in her glass.

'No, my sister does,' he replied, complying with her request.

She asked some more questions, all the time fixing him with those light brown eyes of hers. Robin got caught up in the conversation, so much so that when Janet came to tell him she was leaving, he said he'd get a cab home later. By then Robin felt quite relaxed, having put away several more glasses of the wine. He was still on the same spot, engaged in a lengthy discussion with the woman. Lizzie, as she had told him she was called, had been invited by a friend of hers who worked for the firm. She was a writer she said, lived outside London. When he thought about the evening days later, Robin was quite incapable of recalling what they'd been talking about. In any case, he and Lizzie were still there when the party started to fold up. The next thing he knew, they were in a taxi on the way to her house.

'Robin . . . Robin! Get the phone.'

Robin can hear Janet's voice but he doesn't want to answer her. He doesn't even want to open his eyes but she shakes him, forcing him to come back to reality. Robin sighs heavily, blinks as the bedroom light assaults his pupils.

'What . . .?'

'The phone for you, come on.'

He kisses his teeth, tries to turn away, back to his precious sleep.

'What are you doing sleeping so early anyway? Go and take your call.'

Janet won't leave him alone, so Robin gets up and drags himself to the living room. As soon as he puts the receiver to his ear, he knows he should have stayed in bed.

'Robin? Hi, its me . . .'

'Me' is Marlene, calling as she does every Friday evening. The way he feels right now, Robin can't even make sense on the phone.

'Hmmm, what's happening . . .?'

After several minutes of an awkward conversation, Robin finally puts the receiver down. He has lied, told Marlene he doesn't feel well, invented a flu he's supposed to be suffering from. He gets back to bed even more upset for having done that. Yet there's no way he could meet Marlene right now, not in his present state. As he drifts back to his slumber, Robin once again silently curses his relationship with Lizzie.

Of that first crazy night at Lizzie's house, there's not much Robin could remember either. The house in a quiet suburban street impressed him, although it was late at night and he was in a half drunken state. It was big, luxurious with expensive carpets and furniture and lots of exotic ornaments. He couldn't tell Lizzie's age then, and he's still not sure about that now but she had to be around 40. That's what he reckoned anyway. It was the last thing on his mind that night. She poured him another drink, had one herself and put on some music. Then slowly she started on him; teasing him with her fingers, with her nails, her lips, until they both ended up entwined naked on the living room carpet. Later they reached the bedroom upstairs. Although the accumulated effect of alcohol and his own physical effort had started to take its toll, Robin found himself loving this unknown woman again, furiously. The morning after was like waking up after a fight. In fact, it was mid afternoon when he emerged, wondering what in the world he was doing in this huge four-poster bed, in this strange bedroom . . .

Outside looks greyish, cold and forbidding. 'February already,' Robin thinks to himself as he turns away from the kitchen window to sit down, his cup of hot tea in front of him. His arms crossed on the table, he nods.

   The hot tea stings Robin's mouth as he swallows it, hands wrapped around the mug. A long sleep and a hot bath refreshes him, cleanses his mind. 'It's definitely stopping here, right here,' he says to himself. It sounds like determination this time. Twice before in as many weeks he has returned home from a couple of days at Lizzie's house and chastised himself about what he was doing. Robin knows within himself that the whole business has totally disrupted his life in several ways. The thought of Marlene crosses his mind, he frowns. He better call her and sound convincing . . .

The bell rings twice. Robin gets up, remembering Janet's note on the fridge about Danny calling earlier. He opens up, walks back to the kitchen followed by the tall, square-built young man.

'What's happening?'

Danny sits down, looking at his friend across the table. Robin shakes his head.

'I've just woke up more or less.'

'Yeah I know. What about college yesterday, man?'

Big sigh. Robin shakes his head once again. Frowning, he asks, 'How bad is it?'

It's Danny's time to shake his head. 'Mr Bennett wants to talk to you; something about attendance and grades.'

If only he'd made it to college yesterday, everything could have been straightened out. It's half-term now, that means a full week before he can deal with it. Janet's frowning face appears somewhere in his mind. Danny laughs.

'What about Marlene?'

As if Robin needed that! It's like twisting the knife in the wound. 'Don't even mention it. I'm in trouble.' Robin's half smile lacks confidence. He reads from Danny's face that although he's concerned at his plight, as a good friend should be, at the same time the whole thing sounds to him like a particularly funny joke.

'So, what's new?' Danny asks expectantly.

Robin looks at him serious.

'I'm not going back there, no way.' The tone is definite.

'Yeah . . .? When was it? Last week?'

'Okay, I said it before but this time I mean it.'

Danny shrugs. 'Sure, if you say so.'

It upsets Robin to know that Danny thinks he's too weak to resist. After all, they have been 'partners' for years, sharing everything and always supporting each other, even when it comes to women. It's a matter of honour, to stick to the principles they agree upon. That's how it's always been.

'All right, you watch me. I ain't going back,' Robin declares forcefully.

But Danny is vicious. 'What about your clothes?'

There is maybe a second of hesitation. 'She can keep them.' Robin dismissively forfeits the expensive garments Lizzie has been buying for him every week.

Danny still seems dubious. He asks again. 'And the "chopper"?'

A longer pause. The image of an exquisitely crafted heavy piece of jewellery reflects in both their thoughts.

'I'll give it back, I don't care.'

Eyebrows raised, Danny queries. 'So you're going to go back there . . .?'

'I'll call her and meet her,' Robin counters.

Laughing, Danny stretches. Robin decides to slide out of the topic for the time being. It's Saturday morning, the beginning of a week's holiday; not everything can be bad . . .!

'I haven't had no breakfast, let's go to the café.' He gets up.

'Come on then.'

Robin gets ready quickly and the two walk out of the flat.

'They've been asking for you at the club,' Danny says as they cut across the estate. He adds that their martial arts teacher has expressed concern about Robin's absence; he is meant to be in the team for the competition in two weeks' time. 'Those karate guys are tough; you're gonna get beaten up if you're not in shape.'

'I'm gonna make up for it,' Robin says sombrely.

Danny throws a couple of playful punches across his friend's face, a kick that stops just short of his chest. 'No reflexes,' he teases. 'You're in trouble.'

'Oh yeah?' Robin picks up the challenge and the two fence for a minute or two on the pavement, drawing curious looks from passers-by. It's fresh but sunny this morning. Lewisham High Street is already bustling with shoppers as Robin and Danny cross over to the other side. They get to the small café at the back of a mini-cab office. Inside, half a dozen customers are having a late breakfast, chatting and smoking. They order and sit at one of the vacant tables near the counter. The food soon arrives, not much is said until Robin has emptied his plate. He asks for more tea.

Danny steers the conversation back to his favourite topic. 'So, did you tell her you're not coming back?'

Robin wipes his mouth with a paper towel. He winces. 'I tried, but she didn't take it too well . . .'

Danny smiles. 'No? What happen?'

He doesn't seem to care that even the memory of it turns Robin's face serious. 'She started to get all emotional on me, crying and all that.'

'Crying?' Danny interrupts, maliciously interested.

Robin sits back in the chair, scratches the top of his head. 'Yeah man, it was distressing, I'm telling you.'

'Looks like she's in love with you,' Danny remarks suggestively.

'In love? This thing is just about sex. And it's gotta stop!'

'What did she say?'

Robin shakes his head, blows some hair between his lips. 'She gave me her life story. It was really embarrassing, man.'

'So what happen then?' Danny is unrelenting, thirsty for details, action replay.

'The same thing as always . . .' Robin concedes sombrely.

Laughing, Danny tells him, 'You're a stud, you can't help that!'

'Look, this is no joke, okay?' Robin says, looking around as if checking whether anyone is overhearing them. He adds, 'She's probably over twice my age, that's crazy.'

Danny shrugs, looks around as well before coming closer across the table. 'Listen man, that doesn't matter. You give her what she wants, she looks after you. It's a fair deal, ain't it?'

'No, I can't think like that. What do you think I am?' Robin disagrees with his friend's simple logic.

'You told me she wants to buy you a car, right?'

Robin remembers telling Danny that. He looks at his friend. 'You don't understand; this business is getting out of hand. It's like getting paid for sex.'

Danny nods suggestively. 'You know how many guys would love to get a break like that?!'

'Well, I'm not into that. I've got a life to live, you know what I mean?'

'So what you gonna do?' Danny asks as the waitress clears up their plates.

Robin waits until she's gone. 'I've got to make her understand.' As an afterthought, he adds, 'When I told her I couldn't see her no more, she started talking suicide and all that shit.'

'What?' This is definitely exciting stuff for Danny.

'It has gone too far, I shouldn't have gotten involved with her in the first place.'

'That's not what you said first time though.'

Danny's right; after the first night at Lizzie's, Robin had been on a buzz. She had made him feel different. All his thoughts then had been about getting more of the same thing. But today, barely two months later, Robin feels disturbed by the torrid affair. It's like an addiction, like being hooked or something. Twice already he has gone back to Lizzie's with the firm intention of ending it all. And twice his lust, for that's what it boils down to, has gotten the better of him. Who would have thought he would one day feel ashamed of sleeping with a woman . . .!

'Well, it's up to you. Good luck,' Danny says mockingly.

Robin throws him a malevolent look and gets up to leave. They step into the midday winter sun and hang around the busy high street looking at the clothes in the shops. After hesitating for almost ten minutes, Robin walks inside one of the stores and buys himself the denim suit he saw earlier in the week. He feels a little twinge of guilt as he takes the two crisp fifty pound notes out of his wallet and notices Danny's knowing grin.

The sitcom on the television screen isn't getting much attention tonight. Robin watches, seemingly interested but not seeing a thing. He can feel the probing eyes fixed on him. From the couch, the voice comes over, delicate, almost purring.

'Why don't you come and sit here . . .?'

He glances in Lizzie's direction, briefly thinks about answering something but gets back to the TV. The simple gags of the Sunday evening sitcom are loud in the otherwise silent room. The same thought flashes again through Robin's mind, 'I shouldn't have come.' He's been here less than an hour and has made little progress in his 'mission' so far. Determined to make a clean break from the affair, he left home his mind made up about what he was going to say and how he was going to say it. He hasn't even taken off his coat. The black velvet-covered box is there on the coffee table, the expensive bracelet inside. One approach is as good as any other, he thinks. After that things can only get more upfront.

'Robin, why are you doing this to me?'

Sighing, Robin turns towards the woman looking at him,

her hands clasped in her lap. Lizzie looks fine, even when she's upset like now. Robin does his best not to look at her too hard. He knows only too well how things get started every time he comes here. Tonight has got to be the last time he sees her.

'I'm not doing anything to you. I just have to stop seeing you, that's all.' Robin tries to sound firm, as cold as he can.

Lizzie shifts in her seat, takes a sip from the wine glass in front of her. 'You're sure you don't want a drink?'

Robin is sure; he needs to stay totally sober.

'Is it something I've done?'

Robin can't help laughing. 'Something you've done? No, you haven't done nothing.' He waits a little, switches back from the TV screen.

'Look; I've thought about this whole thing. I don't really feel comfortable, you know what I mean?!'

'No, I don't . . .'

He sighs. The fleeting thought of Danny flashes across his mind. 'I mean, you and me, is just about . . . sex, right?!' he says.

The sounds from the television fill the few seconds of silence. 'Why do you say that?' Lizzie shifts in her seat. For the first time tonight there is eye contact between them.

It's Robin's turn to take a little time before he answers. 'Well . . . in the long term it's not going to last.'

'Why not?' Lizzie's staring at him.

That conversation is precisely what Robin doesn't want to get into. 'You know that; I mean, I've got my own plans, I've got to concentrate on college and all that. I don't think I've been doing that since . . . in the last couple of months.'

Lizzie's almost frowning now. 'So you want to leave me because of college? Am I stopping you from studying?'

Robin leans back in the chair, shakes his head. 'It's not just that . . .' Something in his head, a thought just passing. 'You didn't really think it was going to go on for ever, did you?'

'Why not?' The tone is lower, the eyes squinted.

'This is just crazy,' Robin thinks; he can't believe she ever thought that way.

He looks at her. 'I don't want to get into it, okay? Let's just call it a day.'

Lizzie looks away a little while. When she turns back towards Robin the stare is colder. 'You think you can just use a woman like that? It never occurred to you that I have feelings too?'

He can't resist picking up on that. '"Use"? Talk about it! I'm the one who feels used.'

In a way, Robin regrets saying that. After all he only wants to let her know and leave. No need to argue the point.

'Who do you think you are?' Lizzie sounds really upset now. Then she bursts into tears, buries her head in her hands. Deep inside a voice tells Robin to get up and go. He doesn't. Lizzie stops herself, hastily as if she feels embarrassed at losing her composure. She leans over quickly and takes out a tissue from the box under the table.

Robin feels lousy now, wishing he hadn't taken the argument that far. 'Look Lizzie, I don't mean to hurt you, but it's best we stop it now . . .'

'Best?' she interrupts him. 'Best for you maybe, it's not best for me.' She wipes her eyes, continues. 'What am I supposed to do after you leave me?'

He doesn't want to get into that either. 'Whatever you used to do before me, you've only known me a couple of months.' Bad answer . . .

'Oh, so that's it, just like that!'

He gets up. 'Listen, I don't think I want to talk about it any longer. I've got to catch a train.'

Lizzie looks up at him, her eyes intense and hardened by the painful thoughts inside her. She gets up from the couch. There is an instant of silence as the two pairs of eyes lock into each other. Then Robin's shift away. He starts to the right, heading out of the room.

It is as sudden as unexpected.

'You bastard!!'

Robin turns back towards Lizzie as the insult rings out. The full impact of the short but strong woman hits him. Robin takes a couple of steps back, trying to regain his balance, his arms deflecting the blows thrown to his face. Lizzie is swearing at him, unleashing blows aimed for Robin's face but which come short of target.

'Stop! What's wrong with you . . .?' Robin can't believe that this is happening. He's always suspected Lizzie of having a temper, but he didn't expect her to attack him. This is ridiculous!

Meanwhile, crying and swearing, Lizzie grapples with him. Robin suddenly feels a sharp pain in his chin as Lizzie's pointed shoe makes contact with it. He winces, drops his guard for a second . . . The next thing he knows, Lizzie's right hand makes contact, nails first. The scratch stings the skin of his left cheek, forcing him to cry out.

'You bitch!' he shouts. More blows rain down as if Lizzie is spurred on by her success.

It's Robin's turn to get mad now. He feels more upset than hurt, although just to know his face got marked vexes him. Almost by reflex, he parries the next blow from Lizzie and grabs her arm in the same movement, and spins her clockwise. Drawn in, still shouting abuse, the woman plunges forward as Robin twists her arm forcefully. The lock is perfect, almost too perfect . . . The spin sends Lizzie crashing head first into the tall wall unit, the left side of her forehead smashes against the hard wood with a dull sound. Robin lets go of her arm. He realizes, too late, how strongly he has sent the woman crashing against the heavy piece of furniture. He grabs hold of her quickly, tries to stop her fall as she slumps against the lower shelf of the wall unit. Her body is limp. Robin calls her name, stretches her on the thick carpet of the living room. He feels scared all of a sudden, calls her name again but she seems unconscious. Neither does she respond when he gently taps her face. Her eyes are closed. On the left side of her forehead, a gash in the skin, just above the thin eyebrow. Robin looks about him mechanically, then back at the woman lying before him. His head feels empty. Something grips at his stomach like a claw. Through the open door in the hallway, his eyes rest on the telephone, gleaming black on the white marble-top table.

grub

eroica mildmay

She was on one long vile scenic rebound. The big man with whom she had been for several years had become a possessive monster, his hand for appearance's sake just holding hers, but in reality he was crushing her hand bones together like a mad bitter mother with an errant toddler. She had lived in an arena of fear, until she literally ran away from home. To a great feeling of nothing.

The big man was still after her, milling around the outskirts of her life. She was left in a fragmented state of mind. She probably spent too much time looking over her shoulder as a result and too little looking into her future.

Yet, owing to her looks she was not short of admirers. Abstract admiring gestures ranged from little bits of poetry scrawled on paper dropped through her letterbox to a night full of petty insults from one man who apparently expressed love that way. There were older men, who having avoided the baby mummy trap were still foraging for young ladies, falling in love too fast and too easily as time ran out. And there were married men who borrowed a night off from their accountable weeks to talk in wistful terms about sex at her place.

Buffeted in this jostle of declarations she was able however to make one decision. No married men. She was in awe of the family tribe. None of the 'she doesn't understand me' business cut much ice with her. Hearing of babies, generations to come, filled her with trembles. She, a wisp of straw, could not hope to compete with the completeness of a home, especially one whose front door would remain firmly closed to her. The way was only a bit clearer for that decision.

Jonothan was a friend of a friend. Single and earnest. He stopped her on the street for a chat several times as they were to-ing and fro-ing to the local market. Then he asked her out to dinner. Outright dinner, even in the age of equality, still hints at screwsville, especially if there is no specific topic to discuss. But she couldn't afford a restaurant herself and was sorely tempted. She was pitifully poor, having recently given up her job – the big man had made such a nuisance of himself at her workplace, she had no choice. She agreed to dinner telling herself that she was free to walk away at any time.

He arrived on a bitterly cold evening in February to pick her up in a ratty little sports car. She had to try very hard not to laugh as he rang the doorbell, but only managed to reduce the sentiment to a stilted self-conscious smirk as she opened the door.

She was disappointed to find that they weren't going to a meal on their own. He informed her that two journalist friends of his would join them. They trundled past ever-changing but totally similar scenery, like a cartoon townscape, and deposited outside a folksy downbeat restaurant saved by low lighting.

The journalists worked for *The Sun* and *The Mirror*, and had a professional nose for an impending screw. Jonothan seemed to have neatly managed to straddle the inevitability of the evening with the business of the day. Once he had sealed with relish the chance of some venture he was involved with being covered in 'the popular press' he turned to her. All three of them gazed upon her, desired to take her home and nibble on her, a fact they barely disguised. It seemed routine to declare amongst themselves that they all entertained the thought. It seemed to charge them to think of it, whilst Jonothan was, of course, still king of the road.

On the sidelines, and eating quietly like a shy sheep, a soft fluffy victim, it offended her to be closed off from their conversation whilst being the subject of it. Whatever she did, it seemed as if she was in the waiting room, a fact probably compounded by her silence. But their laughs and their bonding over a common consensus was a fearful barrier to surmount and she didn't tackle it. Jonothan paid the bill for everyone in a wide ranging gesture of goodwill, nods and winks all round.

In the car she talked more to retrieve a sense of herself, and in part did so. He invited her back to his flat and she accepted. I can and probably will leave later on, she said to herself with a weak and saddened spirit.

She was beautiful. When he stopped for a second on his doorstep, turned to her and told her so, there was far more reverence in the comment than she could have guessed at. In truth, he had desired her for a long time, constantly pestering a mutual friend to introduce him. She was different, a bit unspoiled, like Polish girls could be. His family were Polish, and holidays in Poland had given him a taste for simplicity in women, which of course he translated to London women as he had no desire to have a Polish girlfriend. All this, she worked out later.

'Shit, I haven't got any wine. I'll dash out.'

'Here, here's some cash.'

He jumped up, punching his pocket for keys. It annoyed her when he refused to take her money, whilst scanning a desk surface somewhere over her head for a tenner he had deposited earlier. It meant the conquest was his and his alone.

He returned with the wine and two slightly smeared wine glasses held in a knuckle cluster. She took the glasses from him and perched them on the erratic carpet surface. It was almost a moment of intimacy. He poured her a large glass of wine and offered her a cigarette.

'I don't smoke.'

He smoked alone, lying prone in front of the gas fire studiously flicking ash on to a glowing chunk of plastic coal. It toppled heavily and landed on the carpet. Behind his prostrate body, she sat huddled against the cold. The heat from the fire was precious and hard to get hold of. Her face glowed like a pumpkin lantern, but her back felt a deathlike chill. There seemed to be a line down the centre of her body clearly marking the two extremes.

'Are you comfy?' he asked, suddenly aware of her predicament. Comfy? Never was she less comfy, if it came to that.

'Yes, um . . . just a bit chilly, that's all.'

'I'll get you a sweater.'

He brought her a damp woollen sack that sat on her back like a carcass. In it, she could smell his smell. It hung amongst the fibres refusing to emerge to encourage her. But as her body warmed up, it crept out to claim her.

An incredible tiredness came over her. She wanted somewhere to sleep without going back out on to the streets to make her way home. She would end up fucking because she couldn't be bothered, when in fact she couldn't be bothered about fucking. The bottle of wine would be a morbid and cheap anaesthetic to mask her feelings. Her fatigue came over as languidness. He watched closely and wondered when to strike.

When he eventually leaned forward to kiss her, she was more concerned with the wine glass that he nearly knocked over with his knee than with his kiss. He moved it perfunctorily so she could find no further distraction in it and pressed on with his kisses. Everywhere but the lips. Her mouth carefully whispered ahead of his attempts. He accepted this as a game and peppered what part of her face he had access to with butterfly pecks. His hand found her breast but her nipple jangled in his grasp. She had visions of her nipple being rubbed clean away in a plasticine ball and rolling under a chair to gather hair. The image wouldn't clear.

She touched him, moving her hand down along his back, to read him, not to embrace him. There was no play in her. His penis was not a friend, it was simply a member of the public. She did not seek it out.

She managed to drink another large glass of wine between bouts, and was disappointed when the bottle emptied to a last red sip.

He ploughed on with intent, casting brief glances at her to make sure she seemed with him. She did, and that was enough. He feasted on her as the lion does, burying his head in a gazelle to gorge himself. Instead of being freed by it, she feared its intensity and indeed felt like a gazelle succumbing to an untimely death. It nevertheless prepared her in part. She pulled away.

'Let's go to your bed.'

He looked stunned. Interrupted. But he was happy to please her, so he gathered up his sharpened tool, and lolloped into the bedroom.

She just wanted to lie somewhere comfortable so she could sleep.

She stood in the middle of his cold room, unfamiliar surroundings that would steep her in intimacy. The pile of unworn boots like frozen rocks in the corner. His shirts hanging on wispy wire hangers which clung on to the wardrobe door in a particularly gnarled communal grasp. They made her feel sick, and she wanted to snap one off at the neck.

He bent down to light the gas fire. It boomed into the bedroom almost eclipsing his hand in a rounded, domestic and perfectly proportioned fire ball. He pulled his hand back in a flash of anger and looked to see if he had any hair still left on his hands. More or less intact, he walked towards her apologizing for the mess.

On the bed she turned her back to him so she didn't have to look at him. He accepted, a little puzzled. He held on to her thinking, beyond pure pleasure for a second, what a lovely creature she was as she sloped away from him. Her hands on the pillow, her hands spread across his bed, and her lovely smooth behind. He wanted to bundle her up for a moment in his arms, squashing her breasts in a clumsy loving armlock, avoiding their sensuality in a big bear hug of total devotion. A signal of all the times he had watched her passing, and wanted just to speak to her and have her speak back.

Instead he glided along inside her, twitching to find depth. It meant almost nothing to her. His testicles swung heavily against her in a routine patter. She reached out for the headboard to steady herself. He watched her hand hold on firmly and braced himself for the anticipated end.

Afterwards he stroked her hair. She quickly stopped him by putting her hand over his. He left her alone, and slept easily. Granted peace, she couldn't sleep. Instead she lay for a long time looking at the unfamiliar bedroom, the man's mess, his life, his tastes, and felt totally bereft of happiness. She fell asleep on a tear which gathered in her eye but refused to budge until she finally closed her eyes.

She didn't sleep long. She awoke to the smell of a pungent livid fart. A cloud of pure vegetable gas hung like a shroud in the sleeping boudoir. It was poisonous. Is that me or is that him? – she asked herself, doubting that she could produce something so alien to her. She lifted the duvet off her like a thief and left the bedroom. She glanced back at him, despising him for sleeping like a baby through it.

She stood at the top of the landing and looked out of the window. Dawn barely revealed damp railway banks covered by a tangled awning of weeds and, beyond that, puttering trains full of slumped crash robots winding their way into the city. She dressed in cold clothes, and went down to the still kitchen. The windows were slightly misted up which bemused her as there seemed to be no heat source. She found a clammy coffee jar parked in an empty cupboard. The kettle was a whistler, appropriate for a house situated beside the railway. Once the kettle had only half-boiled she made a lukewarm coffee. After one unsavoury sip she tipped it away and put the mug back how it was.

She left, careful to pull the front door closed with the minimum of noise. Out into the suburban chill, freshly bare from folks' nightly retirement into their lace nests.

He did not wake. He slept alone most nights, so he was quite happy lying in his bed as his recent lover made her way through the fading night towards the first pickings of public transport. Through reams of cars shouldered into the kerb for the night. Walking on sugar-coated frosty pavements. She cast her eyes down. A selection of shit-brown leaves and dog shit merged into one crystalline cake decoration. Yum. Yum. No thank you.

When he woke he was hurt. Ghastly. He thought it unfair, sneaking out like that. It rewrote the night before.

She proved hard to track down. She was still dodging the big man, and others. And him.

He presented her with a gift some two weeks later when at last he was able to engineer a spontaneous meeting on her doorstep. He had had five hundred plain business cards made with her name on. Smack in the middle in Roman capitals – SELINA they said, five hundred marvellous times. She looked touched, but not grateful. Remembering her manners she thanked him and went indoors.

the
backwards car

christopher rawlence

The chrome and corduroy chair creaks slightly as the client changes his position. Its empty twin faces him from a short distance across a worn brown carpet. Spring sunlight floods the attic room, emphasizing the grubby white paintwork that's mottled with water stains and the large crack in the ceiling that starts by the light rose and meanders towards the wall.

The client sighs a grey sigh. Metallic breath flows across his furred tongue, through gaps between teeth long worn down by nightly grinding on the secrets that litter his dreams. Today's the day. No going back now on what has to be declared and revealed.

He stares out of the window, through imperfect glass that imbues the bright day beyond with a shimmering sadness. Two men are fitting a television aerial to a chimney stack on the roof of the house opposite. One is stripped to the waist, a slim but muscular Adonis. The other wears a torn tee-shirt with the fading word SEX printed on it. Ripples in the window pane lend their movements graceful fluidity. SEX shakes an arm, sending a wave down a length of cable to free it from where it has snagged on the gutter. Perhaps it's his whip, the client muses, and he's a ringmaster.

The sound of a footfall on the stairs makes him jump. The door handle clinks and the bottom edge of the stripped-pine door snatches at the carpet as Sandy returns to the room with two mugs of tea and a packet of Ritz crackers on a tray. He sits down with a grin, puffing slightly from the longish climb up from the kitchen.

The whistled first line of 'Fly Me to the Moon' drifts across from the aerial fitting operation over the road. A minute passes and neither man speaks. The client feels the weight of the silence, but fears that anything he might say will sound forced and trite. The lack of communication makes him restless, so he reaches for a dirty aluminium ashtray at the foot of his chair and wanders over to the mantelpiece, where he places it next to a bronze Kali. Anxious to fill the awkward lacuna between them, he scrapes his finger-nails across the sooty bobbled surface of the ashtray and launches into a tirade of words: 'Hey, You, with the twinkling blue eyes, I've a question to ask. Why've you given me an ashtray today when you know I'm not smoking? I told you last week that I would not have a cigarette.'

Sandy says nothing. He's used to these aggressive opening ploys.

'You're trying to tempt me,' the client warns. 'You want me to succumb, but I'm not going to. I had my last on the way here. I'm going to face my ordeal without cigarettes.'

Sandy munches a cracker and stares at the client from the lopsided position that he has found most comfortable for his gangly frame over the years. Crumbs litter his straggly beard.

'It's time you bought some new chairs, Sandy.' The client indicates the snatched corduroy fabric of his seat. 'See how creased it's become from the writhing bottoms of all your miserable patients.'

Sandy smiles at the rigmarole of mild insults. He pulls a handkerchief from his pocket and takes off his glasses to clean them. His blue eyes look strange without the heavy frames and thick lenses.

'How many bottoms, I wonder?' the client continues. 'And what stories have their owners confided to you?'

Sandy looks at his watch and lets out an exaggerated yawn.

'Let me put it another way,' the client persists. 'Without specs you look surprisingly vulnerable. It's occurred to me that you must have feelings when we open our hearts to you. Today I find myself wondering how we affect you and how our stories compare.'

The client sits down and takes a sip of tea. 'Am I more interesting than most, for instance? Do you look forward to my visits more than others? Do I particularly fascinate you?'

Sandy averts his eyes. The electric whine of a milk float drifts up from the street. Bottles clink as it comes to a halt. A milk crate hits the step and the doorbell rings, making the client jump and splash tea on the carpet.

'I hope it won't stain,' he says, leaning over the arm of his chair to look down at the floor, where the brown spillage resists sinking in to the tight weave. A tiny bubble floats on it, staring back up at him like an admonitory eye. 'It's watching me,' the client mutters, reaching down to puncture the delicate surface tension that prevents the puddle's dispersal into the carpet.

Taking a tissue from a box on the floor, he rubs away at the spilt tea, then squeezes the dripping mess into a ball which he presents to Sandy in his open palm. 'Looks like a flower, doesn't it. My sad besmirched flower. So knotted and unhappy. See, it's weeping, Sandy.'

A dribble of tea trickles along the client's life line to his index finger, where it merges with the sweaty whorl of the tip. He scrutinizes it closely and says, 'My finger tip's screaming, Sandy. Like an Edvard Munch painting.'

The doorbell rings again and Sandy stands up. 'I should go down and pay him,' he says apologetically. 'I'll only be a few minutes.'

The prospect of the therapist's departure fills the client with unease. *What if he doesn't come back?* he wonders. *I might have left everything too late.*

'Wait a moment,' he implores, 'I've got something for you.'

Sandy hovers at the door as the client fumbles in the side pocket of his jacket. 'I've brought you this to read,' he says, handing Sandy a few scruffily folded pages of typescript.

The therapist leaves the room and the client's unease edges into panic. It's not Sandy's absence he now fears, but his return, when he'll feel compelled to carry out the plan. Feeling suddenly weak, he slips from the chair and crawls across the carpet to a foam mattress that Sandy has laid out in the corner and slumps down. The sun-filled room appears distant to him and its perspective assumes strange angular distortions. He buries his face in the mattress to blot out the bright light. As he lies there, mouth half open against the man-made fibre, he becomes aware of a sickly sweet smell. Raising his head a few inches, he makes out a brown smudge of chocolate melted into the fabric. He lowers his nostrils over the sticky patch. The smell is repellent yet something intimate about it compels him to sniff again. A cluster of memories lurks in the nausea, nudging him gently for acknowledgement. He drifts through a forgotten constellation of feelings that seems to have a bar of cheap strawberry-flavoured chocolate at its centre. The nasty monolith of confectionery commands respect and insists that he smell it.

'Are you my ringmaster, Sandy?' he mumbles. 'Will my performance be just for you or is there an audience out there?'

Five year old Bollock had long blond hair and was sometimes mistaken for a girl. Confusion became crisis one damp June day in 1950, when the natural curiosity of the other kindergarten boys turned into teasing and taunts.

It began in the playground after lunch, when Bollock found

himself unaccountably excluded from the customary huddle round the drain cover. Edward Flagg was the ringleader. 'Are you a boy or a girl?' he sniggered. Bollock was uncertain. 'I think I'm a boy,' he said and everyone laughed. A little later, the question became a victimizing assertion. 'He's got long hair! He's a girl!' they all chanted from the brick box and Bollock found himself crying. His tears made it worse. 'Cry baby!' they sang, and for some reason the teacher didn't stop them.

The cathedral spire loomed spiky and black as Bollock snivelled down the kindergarten path clutching his mummy's hand late that afternoon. He found it hard to explain what was wrong, because until that day he had been unaware that gender held any significance.

'They called me a girl,' he blubbered, and stepped off the kerb into a puddle that had formed in one of the many potholes that scarred the neglected post-war road surface.

'Do look where you're going!' his mother, whose name was Ruth, snapped. She was pregnant and tired, not at all in the mood for whining.

Just then, a shiny black car drew up and distracted Bollock from his misery. It was new and belonged to Edward Flagg's parents. Bollock had noticed it every afternoon that week and was intrigued by the way its flat boot stuck out at the back almost as far as its flat bonnet protruded ahead. In fact, the prominent rear end could easily be mistaken for the front. Did this mean, Bollock puzzled, that the car could move just as effectively in either direction? And if this was the case, what of his grasp of the concept Forwards, which in the brief development of his own motor skills had been associated with far greater speed and agility than his cumbersome experience of Backwards?

Bollock's confusion over the primary orientation of the car

had led him to name it. 'There's the Backwards Car again,' he said to Ruth, as they headed off into the rain.

'Excuse me!' a fruity voice called, as mother and son headed off into the rain. Ruth turned and saw the large figure of Mrs Flagg in a black fur coat emerging from the Backwards Car.

The Flaggs lived in a large mock Tudor house a few miles out of the town. Mr Flagg was a successful stockbroker and commuted to London. They had a swimming pool which they had invited Ruth to use whenever she wanted, but she had been wary of taking up the offer because she did not want to appear dependent on people so much more affluent than she and her husband Michael, who was a farmer.

'May I give you a lift?' Mrs Flagg offered. She wore maroon lipstick on thin lips and pencilled her eyebrows in a Dietrichish kind of way that Ruth found a bit tarty.

'I think we can manage, thank you very much,' Ruth said, with stiff smile.

But Mrs Flagg was insistent. 'It's raining. You'll get soaked,' she said, and Ruth politely capitulated.

The prospect of travelling in the Backwards Car overrode Bollock's dread at having to share the journey with his tormentor, Edward Flagg. As soon as they got in, both boys knelt on the back seat to look out of the rear window.

'Which way will it go?' Bollock asked.

'Forward, stupid,' Edward Flagg sneered.

'But which way is Forward?'

'Anthony doesn't know the difference between Forwards and Backwards, mother,' Edward Flagg crowed. 'And he doesn't know whether he's a boy or a girl.'

The taunt brought the day's ordeal flooding back to Bollock. He felt the press of tears and turned away from Edward Flagg to conceal them. Beyond the high backs of the front seats, his mother and Mrs Flagg were silhouetted against the windscreen, chatting. The rain had become heavier and he could hear the hard patter on the car roof above their voices. The wipers slapped to and fro and Bollock wished that they would wipe his eyes as effectively as they were dealing with the downpour outside.

Mrs Flagg let out the clutch and the Backwards Car lurched forwards. 'Anthony must come round and play with Edward,' she announced. 'The pool's empty at the moment, but there's a water tank that Edward likes to splash in.'

'I'm sure he'd love to.' Ruth turned, expecting her son's excitement, but to her surprise found him staring vacantly ahead. 'Wouldn't you, Anthony?'

Bollock didn't reply. The steady beat of the windscreen wipers had mesmerized him into a fascination with the unfolding view of the street ahead. The decisive movement of the car had cleared up his confusion over its orientation – it was a Forwards Car after all. As it bumped over the uneven road surface, Bollock began to feel that the rounded snout of the bonnet was the questing edge of his own half-formed brow. His delicate sense of boundary expanded outwards to embrace the skin of the vehicle and he felt that he had become the car, that he, Bollock, was splitting the air in front, blazing the trail of the street by prising open the previously solid block of red brick homes.

It was a powerful feeling, and as it intensified, Bollock became aware of a hot pressure inside the front of his cotton shorts. Slipping a hand past the elasticated top, he discovered that his penis had become strangely stiff and extended. As he touched it, a thread of awareness leapt from his frontal lobes to the insistent focus between his legs. This wasn't his first erection, but it was the first time he had ever noticed the strange transformation, and it made him curious. What was this puzzling thing? Why had it grown? And what explained the faint ripples of pleasure he felt when he touched it?

'There's a policeman,' Edward Flagg said, and Bollock, who as yet knew no shame, clambered back on to the seat, with his hand still inside his shorts, to gaze through the back window at a rapidly diminishing local constable on his bicycle and the dark spike of the cathedral spire which seemed to shrink in sympathy with his waning tumescence.

The car turned a corner and they left the long street behind. With its passing, Bollock's puzzlement over gender, that he had somehow crystallized around the ambiguous shape of the Backwards Car, resolved into tenuous certainty. With a sadness that he would only much later become aware of, he recognized the fact of his boyhood. The feminine might-have-been that had lingered on through his infancy, long after nature had settled the issue, now slipped into the boy's shadows where it would lurk in his unlived-out psychological domain of Backwards.

A few weeks later, Bollock was invited round to play with Edward Flagg. Ruth took him on the bus and Bollock insisted on sitting on the front seat, upstairs. They rode down long country lanes, where the unpruned lower branches of horse chestnuts knocked against the aluminium roof and hawthorn scraped the thin sides. About half way there, the bus waited on a stop for an unusually long time. Looking down, Ruth spotted the driver and the conductor sharing a cigarette in the bus shelter. 'We're ten minutes ahead of schedule,' the conductor shouted up to her. 'We've to lose time.'

Ruth took a copy of *Reader's Digest* from her handbag to pass the time. It fell open at 'How to Increase Your Word Power' but the article was hard to read because the driver had not turned the engine off and the vibrations of the idling Diesel caused the bus body to shudder. Ruth found it uncomfortable, but Bollock became aware of the same pleasurable stirring inside his shorts that he had felt during the bumpy ride in the Backwards Car a few weeks earlier.

His first impulse was to tell Ruth, but an unaccountable inhibition held him back. He slipped a hand inside his shorts, as before, and touched the unsolicited erection. The feel of the hard tissue transformed his desire to confess into a compulsion. Words rose within him. Bollock wavered at the threshold of taboo, then he spoke.

'My Tid's all stiff.'

Ruth heard the crude declaration but said nothing. The word Tid was short for Tiddlywonk, which was her dismissive way of tagging the unmentionable. She was reluctant to talk about sexual things at the best of times, but on the top deck of a bus, within earshot of various locals who knew her, it was out of the question. So instead of acknowledging her son's remark, she pointed down at the conductor who had just tossed his cigarette into the hedge and said breezily, 'I think we're about to go.'

Ruth's evasive denial tumbled Bollock from words into deeds. Before she could stop him, he stood up and pulled out the elastic top of his shorts, exposing his pink little erection with an insistence she could no longer avoid. Blushing, Ruth turned away as if the indignity before her was not happening. She was saved by the conductor, who chose that moment to ring the bell. The bus swayed, catching Bollock off balance, causing him to let go of his shorts which sprang back to hide the precocious organ before anyone else noticed.

'Sit down and shut up,' Ruth said firmly, handing him two squares of chocolate to keep him quiet. They were old and had been bouncing round in the bottom of her handbag. Bollock sniffed them gingerly, then hurled them to the floor. 'Uuugh!' he complained. 'They stink of sweet strawberries.'

The bus rumbled on through the countryside. Bollock noticed that the repellent smell of the chocolate had clung to his finger tips. As they neared the Flagg home he found himself repeatedly sniffing the nauseous odour. Each time he sniffed, his body shuddered in revulsion and he resolved to stop doing it. Yet within a few seconds he felt compelled to sniff again and, with a sense of dread and self-betrayal, raised his sticky fingers to his nostrils.

Mrs Flagg served afternoon tea on a cast iron garden table overlooking the empty swimming pool. Winter winds had eddied dry leaves into the corners of the deep end. Ruth watched as a gardener prepared brushes and cans of light blue paint on a trestle table that he had set up in the shallow end.

'The snag with pools is they require too much maintenance,' Mrs Flagg said, pouring the tea. 'If you're thinking of having one, think again.'

An immaculate croquet lawn stretched away from the pool. Edward Flagg was teaching his guest the rules of the game, but the mallet was too big and when Bollock did manage to hit the ball it veered hopelessly wide of the mark.

'I'm bored of this. Let's play in the water tank,' Edward Flagg said, and headed off across the grass towards a rose walk that marked off the main garden from a walled vegetable garden beyond.

'Wait for me,' Bollock called. Ruth watched her small son trail after the spoilt Flagg boy, two small figures in swimming trunks.

The water tank sat alongside a neglected greenhouse that backed up against the south facing wall of the vegetable garden. It was filled by the run-off of rain water from the glass roof, where many panes were broken or missing. A railway embankment overlooked the place, infringing a seclusion that had once boasted a patchwork of annually rotated brassicas, roots and legumes, but now, with the exception of a few rows of lettuce going to seed and a small patch of potatoes, was a riot of dandelions and bindweed.

'Let's take our trunks off,' Edward Flagg said. 'It feels nicer that way.' It was tricky clambering into the tank and, once in, Bollock was wary of the sludge on the bottom that oozed between his toes. The water came up to his nipples and was green with summer algae, and warm.

'What are those squirmy things?' Bollock asked Edward Flagg, who leant back proprietorially against one side, arms outstretched along its hefty rivetted edge.

'Mosquito larvae,' he said, but Bollock was none the wiser.

'Do trains come by here?'

'Of course they do, stupid. Do you like peaches?' Edward Flagg reached up for a furry green fruit that hung over the tank from the gnarled branch of an old peach tree that had found its way out of the greenhouse through a hole in the glass.

'Edward!' Mrs Flagg's distant voice carried across the garden. 'Tea's ready!'

'Let's not go,' Edward Flagg whispered, handing Bollock the fruit. 'We can eat these instead.'

Bollock examined the peach dubiously.

'Go on,' Edward Flagg coaxed. 'I dare you.'

Bollock bit cautiously into the hard fruit, then tossed it away. 'It's all sour!' he shouted.

'You're a coward,' Edward Flagg sneered.

Bollock did not know what a coward was, but from Edward Flagg's tone, it was clearly an insult.

'Only girls are cowards,' the boy continued. 'So you're a girl.'

'You're a girl,' Bollock countered.

'I'm not and I can prove it,' Edward Flagg triumphed, using another strange word that was unfamiliar to Bollock. 'You can feel if you like.'

Edward Flagg took Bollock's hand and guided it down beneath the water surface. 'See,' he said. 'Girls don't have these.'

Bollock was surprised by the jolt of pleasure he felt when he touched the other boy's penis. It was hard, just as his had been on the bus and was once more becoming.

'Mine goes like that too,' he said.

'Prove it,' said Edward Flagg, using the mysterious word again.

Bollock said nothing. He was puzzled about what *proving* entailed and was reluctant to ask. Edward Flagg took his silence as an invitation. His touch triggered a starburst of conflicting emotions in Bollock. He wanted to surrender to the boy's caress yet have mastery of it. He wanted to leave the overgrown place of transgression yet remain there. He wanted to hide the rude secret from his mother, yet describe it to her. He had a powerful sense that the innocent pleasure he had embarked on was wrong, yet had no inkling of why it should be so. He found himself caught at the still fulcrum of a possibility, at which, unknown to him, he faced a choice between two utterly different life journeys.

'Let's touch them together,' Edward Flagg urged. Bollock conceded warily, but had already begun to distance himself from the imminent act. As they rubbed the small swollen tips of their cocks together, bumping foreheads in their eagerness to see into the soupy murk of the water tank, Bollock felt part of himself break away float upwards above the walled garden, where he hovered at a safe distance from the goings on below.

Bollock circled on thermals generated by pleasures snatched by someone other than himself. Scanning the landscape beneath, he spotted a white line of steam edging towards the Flagg property and wanted to cry out a warning. But it was too late, and neither boy heard the clanking approach of the 5.15 from South Godstone, nor noticed the nosey faces of several passengers peering down at two small boys, half submerged in an old water tank, front to front, doing something dubious to each other on a warm June afternoon at the watershed of the twentieth century.

Lying on his back, on the mattress, the client soars above the uneven ceiling of his boyhood. But the tug of the present calls him down. The railway track surrenders its identity to the mundane line of flex that hangs from the light rose. A river, running alongside it, is reclaimed by the meandering crack in the plaster.

A human hair has found its way into the corner of his mouth. The client traces it with the tip of his tongue as muffled voices downstairs intrude on his story. The front door slams. The milk float whines on down the road isolating the sound of someone trying to start a car, its battery weakening from the thwarted effort of coaxing a sluggish engine into life.

The client dislikes the drab actuality of the room. He wants to postpone the nagging summons of consciousness and dwell in his reverie a while longer. Clasping his hands behind his head, he half closes his eyes and blurs the textural insistence of the ceiling so that he can follow the river upstream to its source. He navigates past the brown stains that suggest a loose slate, to the wall where the river elbows down towards the mattress, narrowing to a hairline as it passes his head before vanishing behind the skirting.

Sandy's room slips away again. The walls take on a purplish hue and vertical wooden bars prevent him rolling off the mattress. Something's missing. Lying there on his back, the client is struck by an absence. He has woken to an early spring afternoon, expectant, alert, knowing only that whatever has deserted him should shortly be making its reappearance.

Every sound holds significance as the client strains his ears for some trace of the absent thing, but it does not return. He shifts his gaze to the stains in the ceiling which mutate into faces, each expressive of particular emotions. Curiosity leads his eye across a flaky montage of love, compassion, sadness, anger. A tiny fire starts where their feelings impinge on him. Its heat is intermittent and appears responsive to the emotional field of others. Baby Bollock smiles as the first flashes of self bounce between his disparate levels of awareness, then frowns as a pervasive and real heat floods his nappy.

The creaking tread of a stair alerts him. A familiar shape moves in his peripheral vision. His perceptions and feelings unite into a snatch of consciousness as she towers above him and smiles down into the cot. She lifts him out and he nuzzles in the milky hollow of her neck, but before he has time to feel safe again, he is thrust on to a rubber mat where she removes the sodden towelling and leaves him cold and exposed, legs flailing, to wander over to the cupboard.

A dog's whine filters up from downstairs. Sharp smells of urine and rubber envelop him. She returns with a largish white object which clanks when she puts it down on the floorboards. His head falls back as he feels himself lifted into an enforced sitting position on a strange seat with a circular lip that digs into his bottom. He struggles to get off but is commanded to stay put in tones he knows must be obeyed.

Bollock sits on the potty, wanting approval for an indeterminate task. His mother knits in the chair opposite and ignores the repeated whining of the dog downstairs.

Sandy munches a segment of orange and watches the client from his chair. The client rolls away from him and says, 'Oh, it's you, back again. How long have you been gone?'

'A few minutes. Have a piece of orange.'

'I think I need to piss,' the client replies. He hauls himself shakily to his feet. The journey to the door seems unending and he finds the resinous smell of stripped pine on the landing overpowering. He lingers outside the toilet door, allowing himself to be waylaid by the pattern of the woodgrain in its panels. The linear swirl recalls the sad whorl of his finger print and suggests the furrowed undulations of a worried brow.

Once inside, he closes the door behind him, lifts the seat, and fumbles with his fly. The white bowl looks up at him from far below. Its tiny stretch of clear water invites the foaming violation of his urine stream. He signals the release of the appropriate muscle, but nothing happens. He tries again and realizes with a shock that he is unable to let his piss go. The muscular complex that serves his pissing and shitting has seized up in stubborn paralysis.

Panic grips him. He feels suddenly vulnerable from behind. It's not so much his back that feels exposed as his arse. Letting his piss go will also entail releasing his anal sphincter, thereby opening his arsehole to unpredictable possibilities. It's not the humiliation of shitting himself he fears but the unsolicited entry of something or someone into him.

The client holds his breath and listens. He has the strong sense of someone standing behind him, but when he turns there is only the closed door and the swirling reprimand of the woodgrain. He tries to piss again, without success. Terror displaces panic as he contemplates never pissing again.

Once back in the room, the client collapses on to the mattress and the awesome difficulty of the now imminent task presses in on him. Sandy watches him, looking strangely like his mother.

'Are you knitting?' the client asks, convinced he has seen the flash of needles.

Sandy nibbles the end of his stainless steel ballpoint. 'Just taking the odd note,' he replies.

'I can't piss,' the client says.

'What's holding you back?'

'I shouldn't have drunk all that tea.'

He buries his face in the mattress in a vain attempt to smother his mounting distress, but the darkness that encloses him brings no relief. Instead, he feels the rise of an asphyxiating repugnance in his chest. He turns violently on to his back and gasps for breath. He stretches, then curls up into a foetal position. He thrashes from side to side, in an attempt to ward off the inevitable, but no conceivable bodily configuration offers him a way out.

'How long does it take a boy to drown?', the client whispers. His agony brings back warning stories of those who went swimming too soon after lunch and were caught out of their depth by paralyzing cramp. And tales of air-beds swept out to sea by treacherous currents, found two days later with no trace of their young occupants. How did these children die, he wonders? Did they struggle, as he's struggling now? At what point did their resolve to live slide into acceptance of death? When was the threshold crossed, between the physical agony of drowning and that stage at which, it's said, *my whole life passed before me.*

He's heard that it only takes a few minutes to drown, but this is taking an eternity. It's a suffering shot through with the echoes of his mother's disgust. Aaaachh!, she goes, at the cowering black and tan dachshund that has pissed on the living room rug. Bad boy! Aaaachh! she repeats, rubbing the nose of the poor animal forcefully in its mess. Aaachh! she shouts, relishing the glottal stress of the sound as she projects her own sense of shame on to the humiliated animal.

The punishing sound resounds up the winding staircase of the client's formation and locks on to his bewilderment at why he is sitting there on the potty. Her curses reverberate from the walls of the attic room where he writhes on the floor. 'I will die. I will . . . there's a word I can't find . . . I will . . . I'll . . .,' the client moans, but the word eludes him.

The moment is upon him and nothing can now stop him. He rolls over on to his back and looks Sandy straight in the eye. With his right hand he pulls down the top of his tracksuit trousers and says, 'I'm going to show you my cock.'

Sandy doesn't flinch, but neither does he look at the smallish flaccid thing that the client is exhibiting with so much effort.

'Why don't you look at it?' the client demands.

Sandy lowers his eyes to the wrinkled hairy place. 'I've got one of those too,' he grins. 'But I'm not going to show it to you.'

'I've not finished,' the client says. 'I have something to say to you.'

He lifts his trunk clear of the mattress and eases his tracksuit trousers down to his knees. Turning over into a crawling position, he lowers his chest to the mattress and faces Sandy with his splayed exposed arse. 'I want you to fuck me,' he murmurs into the sweet surface of the mattress. 'Fuck me please, Sandy.'

It is shown. It is said. Leaden tension drops away from the client, freeing him to spin in a place of soft caressing pinkness. For an hour he remains in the vulgar vulnerable position. Now and again the sound of Sandy moving in his chair punctuates the benign chorus of redemption that sings through him.

An ice cream van on the street finally levers him back into the room. He lifts his face from the mattress to the melody of a truncated 'Greensleeves'. A ray of evening sun imbues the bronze Kali on the mantelpiece with an orange glow. He pulls up his trousers and turns to face Sandy.

The client feels no shame and Sandy holds his gaze, acknowledging that what's just happened is no everyday occurrence in the white attic room, where souls are bared more frequently than arses.

'Have you ever wished you had breasts?' the client asks, cupping his hands under the flabby pectorals beneath his tee-shirt. 'Wonderful proud tits that you could flaunt at me?'

Sandy raises an eyebrow. 'Not me,' he says. 'But perhaps they'd suit you.'

The client moves his hands to cover his collarbones, protecting his chest with crossed arms. 'I'm still searching for that word,' he says, rocking gently backwards and forwards. 'It's on the tip of my tongue.'

A little later he finds himself once again towering above the lavatory bowl. The seat is still up from his last thwarted attempt. He pulls out the innocent looking tag of flesh and waits, but this time release comes easily. A silvery stream of piss arcs down towards the water. The bubbly tone of its fall resonates from the white porcelain, a hollow archetype of sound that evokes the essence of physical relief. He looks down. Foam covers the surface which seems to have taken on a pink tinge.

Still pissing, the client stoops to take a closer look. The pink is unmistakably deepening into a visceral red and his piss stream has turned crimson. 'I'm pissing blood,' he says to himself.

'Pissing blood,' he repeats, surprised at his lack of concern, relishing the continuing ebb of a tension that he wishes would go on for ever.

'Surrender!' he says abruptly. 'That's the word!'

The urine keeps flowing, redder and redder, and a delicious sense of release spreads through his abdominal region. The clenched button of his anus petals outwards like trusting labia. He lets go the uptight musculature of ejaculation. The sensation is as much an embrace of the idea of being fucked as it is a preparedness to expel or give birth to something inside him that is demanding release.

He looks down at his penis. The piss slows to a puce drip as if inhibited by a blockage within. As he watches the veined stalk in his hand, he notices a strange swelling at its root. It looks like the knotty ball of a dog's prostate that curiosity led him to fondle on the stiff penises of his boyhood pets. But in contrast to those canine hard-ons, this swelling appears to be edging towards the tip of his cock, like the half-digested body of a lamb in a python's gut.

He searches his anatomy for the contractile muscles that might help to expel the strange lump, but can find none. He need not have bothered because the lump finds its own way along his stretched urethra. He watches in amazement as a bloody bolus of shreddy tissue the size of a golf ball pushes out from the tip of his penis, like some gruesome egg, and tumbles down into the bowl with a splash.

He turns away. An old Dinky toy on the window sill catches his eye. It's a battered model Studebaker from around 1950 that looks surprisingly like the Backwards Car. He tucks his cock back inside his fly and picks the car up. Its tyres are hard and cracked, and the blue enamel paintwork is badly chipped, revealing a dull grey diecast body beneath.

He puts the toy back on the sill and drives it up and down between a roll of toilet tissue and a new box of Tampax. The noise of the wheels resonates inside the body with a tinny note he can almost hum. This way and that way he drives, forwards and backwards, with the confidence of a driver who can now navigate just as easily in either direction.

He looks down into the bowl again. White foam surrounds a yellow island of urine. There's no sign of the malignant lump he just ejected, nor any trace of red.

'Serenity was the word,' he whispers to himself, triumphantly. 'Not Surrender.'

according to michael

evelyn conlon

Once upon a time, that is last year, two women drank coffee in Bewleys of Grafton Street, and tried to talk everything off three years, tried to hint things together chronologically, to overview events, to swim people and their actions and their intentions in and out of the stream. Gossip it's called. They did this because it said their lives out to each other and thus made them seem more understandable.

There had been a long six months, fifteen years before, when they had come here every Saturday, them and their pleased crowd. They had small breakfasts, lots of coffee and cinnamon buns. They had read their *Irish Times* and been widely envied because everyone could see that they were it that year. A small group of lucky people who could have been the cloud in *Les Idées claires*, according to Michael. He would have said that, he was the only art student in their crowd. They rarely understood his references.

But the stone moved on top of them and in some cases hit off the cloud. There was tragedy and failure as well as contentment and dizzy success. The most unexpected rose to the top, the most unexpected slid to the bottom. Some of them married others of them, some of the women married farmers, (no fear of that for our two in Bewleys, they were farmers' daughters and knew better). Some married and separated with indecent suspicious haste, some lingered through years. Many emigrated and added that particular sweet and sourness to their lives. Barbara was one of those, now living in Boston.

'I'm glad it's all over,' Barbara said, referring to sexual desire, 'it was a thing that could drive you mad.'

She said she hadn't felt an urge, an uncontrollable one, for more than a year.

'And what did you do if it was uncontrollable?' Sadhbh* asked, them not having the legal language to imagine any action suited to that sort of predicament nor indeed the stories that admitted it. Barbara dithered, in a confident way, and mentioned self help, using her own hand with the assistance of thoughts that she'd have sworn were crazy if anyone had written them down claiming them to be normal.

'But mostly,' she said, 'I went to pubs or night clubs, got drunk, very drunk, and found a man.'

'Why did you have to get drunk?' Sadhbh asked, thinking what a waste of sensation, although knowing the unfairness of her question.

'If a woman who needs it has not been asked by the second drink she'll get drunk for sure. And then she can ask herself.'

'With all your degrees in Sociology?'

'Those never helped get a man on a dark night,' Barbara said.

But that wasn't what Sadhbh had meant, Sadhbh had meant why would Barbara get so drunk at all, having all those degrees, Masters actually.

Barbara and Sadhbh were different, as most people are. They come, or came, from the same place, a village in County Monaghan. In Ireland you always come from your county even if it be only so many miles by so few. But some people get

---

*–*adhbh*, pronounced as -ive in *dive*.

to say 'came' from. They met and maybe loved each other because of this geography. Actually it was the coming fromness that made them meet, the love was luck and icing.

'Anyway, it's all over now, thank God. That ridiculous hunger has been fed. I hope. What about you?'

'I've never really not enjoyed sex. I think I've been lucky,' Sadhbh said, dodging her terrible secret.

And she recounted again how she'd met her husband, as if they didn't know, and reminded herself and Barbara how placid and almost great her life was, which was a little petty considering everything Barbara had just told her. And untrue.

But she reminded herself later that these three-yearly conversations with holidaying emigrants were too difficult because they raked up comatose and dangerous feelings which were best left hidden. Feelings that were as things which Sadhbh had been looking after, hoping that no one would come back looking for them.

Of course her reply had been only half honest, not because it was half dishonest but because it was wholly half honest. She had after all shut down the truth. It was not something that she liked talking about. Anyway sex and everything with it, love, flirting even, had always come as surprises to her, as extras. Pity, then, that it was not easy to trim her expectations.

In winter time when Sadhbh was young she had never thought that she wouldn't always have to play cards with the old ones at home while her brothers went to dances or just went out. Out where? Out into the dark lane? Or out down the road? But there's nothing down the road. Dances – maybe she could understand that, although she couldn't fit an interest in dancing with her big lolloping brothers, here she was very wrong, unlike most they were not going to dances merely to see people, they were in fact the best jivers for miles around. They spun their troubles into handleable disappointment in perfectly timed circles.

Then one evening she was told that she could go with them. Luckily she too had rhythm so was no disgrace on the floor and never experienced wallflowering, well once or twice but she assumed that was only because someone hadn't got to her on time or hadn't seen her before asking someone else. A few months later she went to the pictures with a man. She had never been before, the nearest picture house being ten miles away. The darkness shocked her but that was soon to be nothing; the man put his arm on her shoulders. Casually, loosely. It took Sadhbh all of a long quarter minute to realize what the weight was. It was so dark she thought that something might have fallen on her shoulder. When the truth dawned on her a nausea never before experienced came over her body, her stomach sprouted troughs and she thought she would faint. The man must have felt the rigor because he excused himself. While he was gone she wondered should she run away but how would she get home? She knew no one in this town. She didn't even know the road out of it. He came back with a box of Roses chocolates and didn't put his arm near her again. She would have liked to eat one of the chocolates in gratitude but her tongue was stuck to the roof of her mouth and stayed there for hours even after he had left her home, even after she had thrown the chocolates into the cooker. The poor man. Never had such hatred been felt for such a small gesture.

Sadhbh protected herself from privatized encounters with boys for a long time after that, but then, unknown to herself, she became ready and fell into casual dating with a boy who was the same age as herself. Her first kiss was a surprise rather than a thrill, the second was distasteful, the third was more than satisfactory. In time the two of them negotiated a lying down beside each other in a field, and she had an astonishing clothes-on, little-touch, just-weight orgasm. Thus did the geography of her sexual life begin.

'Sadhbh Quinn, find the source of the river, and trace it to its outlet.'

'Yes, Miss.'

'No, the Shannon does not start in Limerick, it starts in Sliabh Cuilcagh in Cavan, it ends in Limerick. There's a difference between a beginning and an ending. You know that Sadhbh, I presume.'

Indeed she did. She was well acquainted with the ending, the ending of life, with its inevitability, its importance, indeed there was a continuous effort being made to make sure that she never forgot it, and prepared herself for it well. Why only last month Mickey Larmer and James Linden had crashed into each other going around a corner over the road, James Linden shouldn't really have been on their road because it could hold only one car, he should have taken the main road. It was so close. The rosary beads in Mickey Larmer's pocket were crushed and there wasn't a scratch on him. He could have been killed. He should have been killed, they said, their voices rising hysterically. Sadhbh exchanged 'nearly was' for 'should' in order to get to the root of the hysteria. And they marvelled at how two cars would just happen to meet on a blind corner over the road exactly when the hedges had overgrown wildly, the holes in them casting bright shadows across the road, so bright they would take the sight away from anyone's eyes. And how when that did happen nothing more serious had to be done than mend the doors, put a lick of paint on them and buy a new pair of rosary beads. Oh! yes, you had to stay on the side of God.

'How does the source of a river begin, does it start with a drop of rain or what, Miss? And why does the river go one way and not another and why does a mountain rise up where it does and how come?'

'You'll learn all of those details in time, Sadhbh.'

Sadhbh's father and mother taught her about the evil of sex through a series of verbal contortions, intaking of breaths and loud aggravated sighs. They laid down markers so that Sadhbh knew without being specifically told that she was not to go near the New Houses, a County Council estate at the end of the village, where the sexual habits were less rigid than out their road. So who did Sadhbh first really and truly love? A man from the New Houses of course. But they got her to Dublin to a University just in the nick of time, where God alone knew who she'd meet, and all they could do was hope.

During the Bewley's six months Michael asked her to marry him and she told him not to be so silly. She had neither the broad view nor age to help her answer the question in a real way. She told him that you couldn't just ask someone to marry you. Michael persisted and said that you could because you had to start somewhere and there wasn't an infinite number of questions that a person could put before getting down to the important one. But it dawned on Michael slowly that Sadhbh had really refused him, that she wasn't simply playing with him. He had vaguely heard of Mount Isa, Queensland – once – and thought that that should be far enough away.

'I won't be distracted by art galleries there,' he told Sadhbh and said that he'd always wanted to go to a mining town, hadn't he told her? When he was gone a few weeks Sadhbh realized that there is more to a map than the coloured-in mountains. She knew, without knowing, that she had fallen into a bottomless lake. That summer she didn't notice the trees dressing up, or the flowers pollinating all over the place, or the sun showing off.

In time, that being a word that gives some notion of Sadhbh's sense of loss, she married. Her flatmate, Barbara in fact, had convinced her to try wearing a pair of false eyelashes as they dressed for their Saturday night out. Perhaps it was the unexpected heat in the pub corner or maybe she hadn't used the solution properly, whatever, a sensation made itself known to her, that of roof tiles tumbling irresistibly towards the ground. A person can think a lot in a moment like that and Sadhbh saw a woman's pants, at one of the home dances, creep down her legs. The woman stepped seriously out of them and kicked them under a seat in perfect time as if it was all part of the dance. So Sadhbh caught the offending eyelash before it fell into her Guinness, ripped the other one off and popped both of them into her matchbox without missing a beat of her conversation. The man who was listening to her felt a great joy squeeze into his bones. He had to marry her and because Sadhbh didn't know how to refuse twice, they did.

Time was spent, children were born, holidays were had, letters were written, Barbara and others were seen when they came home.

But Sadhbh had not intended to see Michael on his first visit back, she had met him accidentally. She was running in and out of late night Thursday shops too busily when she felt the heat of someone looking at her. When she realized that it was Michael who was stepping towards her with his mouth slightly open she blinked. Her stomach blushed. They kissed on the cheeks quickly. Observant passers-by would have smelt singeing. After ticking off the luggage of their lives, small inconsequential things like spouses, offspring, addresses, wages for bread, years, they made a casual arrangement to have coffee at ten o'clock on Saturday morning. Both of them tried their best to weigh the words with ordinariness but puffs of tunes came into the sentences making a sudden untraceable music heard above the street din. Some people looked around, then told themselves they had only imagined it.

And when that Saturday had happened, when its creation of intimacies had exploded into dusk, the pasts of Michael and Sadhbh had been bloodily stained with unfillable desire. The mistake of finding out would be with them forever.

Michael returned to Australia on Sunday. Sadhbh was sorry that she knew that. She listened for the noise of every plane in the sky.

Since then there was only one certainty. After all the building of a life she knew that there was nothing inside. Every daily task became a falsehood but most of all sex and everything leading to it became a colossal lie. Her husband, who had never done her any harm, seemed to be a torturer. His hands, that were only hands, became objects of fear, his skin became as thorns and she dared not think of his penis because of the terror it held. All bad. All that geography dried up. Memory become an enemy.

'How long ago did this happen, who have you told?' Barbara asked, sadly, when Sadhbh had finally wound herself to the end of her story.

'Two years. No one.'

'Is there nothing you can do?'

'I remember Michael saying that unlike Rodin we can't divide the body into sections and make them pretend that they have nothing to do with each other.'

'He would,' Barbara humphed.

'What?'

'Nothing.'

'After I left you last week, I thought that I should really tell someone. I thought that saying it might make it not be true. I thought that if I told you it might make it easier.'

'And has it?'

'I'll see.'

Barbara wondered if the weight of such a thing could flatten a person, could drag them slowly, prematurely into the earth. And should Sadhbh tell the truth to her husband? And should she go to Mount Isa? Yes indeed, Michael felt the same way as she did but she had begged him not to write again.

Sadhbh dropped Barbara, on her way back to Boston, out to the airport. Barbara said, 'I'll call you at Christmas.' In reply, Sadhbh said, 'An awful lot of planes leave here every day. Go places.'

groupie

john hoyland

1.

'We'll show you a good time,' drawled the voice on the phone. 'And that's a promise.'

Tony thought for a moment. The invitation to go up to Manchester had come as a surprise.

'You don't think we could do the interview now on the phone?' he asked.

'No way, man. If you want to write an article about us, you should come to our gig . . . We'll make it worth your while, I mean it.'

Chas Weymouth, the owner of the drawling voice, was the drummer with a Manchester band called Cuddly Toys. He was also one of the organizers of a music co-operative called Music Matters. Tony had been commissioned to write an article about 'alternative music' for *Rock On*, a music monthly he contributed to. Music Matters was one of the groups he wanted to talk to.

He decided he would go to Chas's gig. His life, he told himself, was far too short on good times at the moment. The prospect of getting away from London for a couple of days was distinctly appealing, and the prospect of getting away from his messed-up marriage even more so.

When he put the idea to Sara, his wife, she agreed to it with almost unseemly haste, even though it meant she would be stuck with the children for the weekend.

Early on Saturday morning, he set out in his green mini-van, and headed up North. Despite the grey winter skies, once he was on the M1 his spirits rose. Most people he knew didn't like motorways (Sara, in particular, often railed against them) but he loved them. He liked the speed, the busy flow of traffic, the sense of everybody on the move. He even liked the service stations, with their trash food and their garish decor and their rows of electronic games with flashing lights and noises of machine-guns and racing cars. He liked observing the people in the tacky restaurants and shops, as wide a cross-section of humanity as you could find, but all temporarily homogenized by the common denominator of travelling.

So he drove up the motorway feeling good, imagining he was a bachelor again, his fantasies roaming about picking up beautiful girl hitchhikers and generally having exotic sexual adventures in the two days that lay ahead.

He coaxed what he felt was a remarkable performance out of the mini, and arrived in Manchester at 4 p.m. It was almost a disappointment to reach his destination. The freedom he had felt on the road gave way to a sense of responsibility about what he was here for – the article he had to write, the people he had to meet and deal with. He took his music journalism very seriously.

He made his way through the city centre, noting how the fine old municipal and financial buildings he remembered from an earlier visit were being busily replaced by blocks of windswept concrete and glass. Eventually, after getting lost a couple of times, he found his way round the ring-roads and drove out to the terrace of run-down Victorian houses where Chas Weymouth lived.

Chas, when he appeared at the door, was a picturesque figure. He had a thin, lugubrious face, made rather menacing by a badly chipped front tooth. His hair was extremely long and greasy, and when he greeted Tony he was wearing a large, shaggy fur coat, despite the gas fire which heated his two-room flat. This flat was as untidy as anywhere Tony had ever seen. It was littered with posters, mattresses, cushions, records, wires, amplifiers, speakers, musical instruments, coffee cups, magazines, stacks of paper and a large, ink-smeared duplicator.

'Is this where you live?' he asked incredulously.

'Sometimes,' said Chas, giving him a lopsided grin. 'It's also the Music Matters HQ. This is where the operation is run from – the nerve-centre sending out pulses of anarchy all over the North of England.'

Music Matters was a co-operative of 100 or so musicians and interested parties who had banded together to form their own management, booking agency and equipment hire service. They were also involved in opening up new venues and promoting local bands. The idea, Chas said, was to cut out the middle-men, and to counter the London domination of the music scene.

Over coffee in the flat's filthy little kitchen, Tony took notes while Chas explained the set-up in an accent that was part Mancunian, part mid-Atlantic hippy. But he finished by saying that he wasn't really 'into' talking.

'I'm just the dumb drummer, you see. The point is to come to the gig this evening. That's where you'll understand it all. Me talking about it's a bit irrelevant really.'

The gig took place in a large, ugly hall that had once been a Methodist chapel. Three local bands were playing, including Cuddly Toys. Driving into the town centre with Chas, Tony noticed that the streets had been well plastered with publicity for the evening.

'When you're putting on your own gigs, you really work to pull the punters in,' commented Chas. 'Not that it's absolutely necessary, because we've already got a big following who turn up anyway. But we always try to bring in new people, to establish Music Matters as a force.'

The three bands turned out to be competent and likeable, without being exceptional. The first was an R&B band from Liverpool who ran through a repertoire of standards that Tony couldn't help enjoying because R&B had been the music he had loved at university ten years earlier. Then there was a satirical outfit who effectively parodied various musical styles and enjoyed a warm rapport with an audience that had obviously seen them several times before. Then Cuddly Toys came on. They played what Tony thought of as Notting Hill rock – a combination of West Coastish psychedelia and heavy metal, with lyrics that dealt exclusively with drugs and fucking. Finally, all the musicians from all the bands came on stage and finished up with an enthusiastic jam.

Quite early on, Tony had decided that though Music Matters was interesting as an organization, the kind of music it promoted belonged to the past. The impression was confirmed by the audience – the large following Chas had talked about consisted almost entirely of unreconstituted sixties hippies, though the year was now 1975. He managed to discuss this briefly with Chas, and Chas agreed that the audience was rather a specialized one. But when Tony probed him further – about putting over positive ideas through the music, or reaching out to new audiences – Chas clearly began to feel a bit out of his depth.

'Well, I'm not against ideas, you know,' he said. 'But most of all I'm into having fun. So long as the punters turn up and have fun as well, I don't really care who they are.'

It was a different attitude from the extreme political earnestness and quest for ideological correctness that dominated Tony's life in London, and for a while he was confused by it. He spent the early part of the evening going round with his notebook, conscientiously trying to make a correct analysis of the occasion for his article. But meanwhile, the bar at the end of the hall was serving excellent Northern beer, and there were lots of attractive girls about, and he made frequent trips to the musicians' dressing room to take drags on the joints being smoked there, and before long he was quite stoned and wondering if Chas's philosophy didn't have something to be said for it after all.

Just before he went on stage to drum in the final session, Chas came up to him and whispered:

'There's a party afterwards. It's going to be good . . . You see, when I told you we'd give you a good time, I meant it.'

During the jam session, Tony watched the people dancing. There was a good-looking girl nearby in tight white jeans and a woolly Afghan coat. She was moving with graceful poise in front of a large, clumsy man who stuck his bottom out and jerked around with a stiff torso and bandy legs. Tony noted, not for the first time, how much better at dancing women were than men. Why was that, he wondered? And why did black people tend to dance better than white people? The truth of these clichés disturbed him.

As for his own dancing, at first he was self-conscious about it. Were people watching him, he wondered? He looked round, half-hoping, half-fearing that they were. He also checked his own dancing against other people's, to see if they danced better than he did. He liked some of the movements a nearby girl in a long, loose, floral skirt was doing, and wondered if he could imitate them – but then wondered if they weren't too feminine for a man to do. He started to worry that the way he danced was maybe a bit effete. If he wriggled his hips in such and such a way, did it look sexy, or did it look silly?

The fact was, he was a lousy dancer, he decided.

His self-consciousness was exacerbated by something else that had bothered him on and off throughout the evening. There were two particularly pretty girls dancing immediately in front of the stage, and he was badly attracted to both of them.

One of these girls was blonde and one was dark. They both wore a lot of make-up and bright, sexy clothes. The blonde, who was the plumper of the two, had a low-cut pink sweater that revealed a disconcerting amount of her breasts, and figure-hugging purple satin pants that left one in no doubt about the precise contours of her bottom and crutch. The dark one was skinnier, with an impish, hungry-looking face and a large mouth. She wore, in spite of the season, a black halter top that left her pale arms, her back and her midriff bare. She also had a tight black skirt with a slit up one side, and black fishnet stockings.

Both girls wore stiletto heels and, when they weren't conferring with each other and giggling, both danced in ways that Tony found highly provocative. He couldn't make up his mind which of them was the more attractive – and, more seriously, he couldn't sort out his response to them, which ranged from ravenous curiosity about them (what motivated them to act out the role of fantasy objects with such evident relish?) to an infuriating sense of inadequacy and deprivation in relation to them. He was quite certain that he lacked the sexual confidence and know-how to approach them.

They seemed to be 'with the band' in any case, as such girls so often were. Various musicians during the evening had winked at them or exchanged a brief word as they played, and at one point Chas himself caught their eyes while he was drumming. He proceeded to stick out his tongue at them and roll it lasciviously round his lips. The girls seemed to find this funny.

Tony wondered which of them Chas was fucking and decided he was probably fucking both of them. He probably fucked both of them at the same time.

His feeling of deprivation deepened. Other people had all the fun. Other people had the prettiest girls, the wildest, most abandoned times . . .

During the jam session the girls noticed Tony staring at them. After he had briefly met the black-haired girl's eyes, she whispered something to her friend, who then glanced in Tony's direction. It seemed to Tony that when she did so, all the fun and lightness left her face.

Saddened and embarrassed, he turned away and tried to concentrate on his dancing again, which now seemed more difficult to get right than ever.

But his awkwardness didn't last long. The massed musicians on the stage were really playing rather well now, and the music was beginning to get to him. In his moments of self-consciousness he had thought of stopping dancing, but he found he couldn't. His body and his mind were getting connected up to the music, and he was beginning to let go, to stop caring what sort of impression he might be making.

It was getting to other people too. He met the eyes of the girl in the floral skirt and their movements temporarily gelled together. He smiled the pleasure he was feeling at her, and she smiled back the same pleasure. Then she turned away, back to her partner. Tony turned away too and got more than ever into the music. He glanced at the two girls by the stage to find they had their backs to him and he didn't have to worry about them knowing he was looking at them any more. He threw himself into his dancing more and more, until he was sweating and his pulse was racing and he suddenly felt innocent and happy.

Chas was right. Having fun was what really mattered. To hell with ideological correctness.

2.

The music ended on a massive discord that went on forever, punctuated by melodramatic crashes of cymbals and drums from Chas. A surprising number of people from the audience stayed on to hump the gear out of the hall into the Music Matters van. Tony helped carry a few things as well, but soon tired of it and went back to the bar to finish his beer.

His mind went back to London. Sara would probably be going to bed round about now, and there was little doubt that she would be going there with her lover.

The fact that she had a boyfriend was the latest in a series of upsets in their relationship over the past few years. Ever since Sara had become a feminist at the end of the sixties (or so it seemed to Tony), their marriage had been riven with discord. They had fought over their responsibilities in the home, over looking after the children, over which of them took jobs and when; they had even fought over the kind of food they ate, since Sara's feminism had for some reason also involved a conversion to vegetarianism. Every aspect of their lives had been examined for its ideological implications, and almost invariably been found wanting. And in the end, because Tony himself took feminism seriously and felt it ought to be supported – and because, in any case, he was obliged to admit that Sara frequently had logic on her side – she had won virtually all the arguments.

Even his few victories had tended to be pyrrhic ones. Taking lovers, for example, had been his idea. All their friends were doing it, and he didn't see why they shouldn't be liberated in this respect as in all the others. But Sara, having initially opposed the idea, had turned out to be much better at having lovers than he was. She was now enjoying a long-lasting and intense romance with a person named Joe, while Tony had only managed a couple of brief and puzzlingly unsatisfying affairs.

He had also found himself much less able to cope with her infidelity than he had expected. He was profoundly thrown by her involvement with Joe. But since jealousy was regarded as an incorrect emotion at the time, and since he had proposed the idea of having an open marriage in the first place, there wasn't a great deal he felt he could do about it – except to snipe at her and sulk and make it clear that he considered he was very hard done by, a notion that she strenuously resisted.

Taking lovers, in other words, had done nothing to improve their rocky relationship.

Well, he was glad to be out of it for a while, glad to be here in Manchester, free and enjoying himself. He took things far too seriously in London. He was entitled to a bit of pleasure for a change.

The party was in a bare, sparsely furnished flat that, judging by its ancient and hideous wallpaper, had only just been purchased by its new owner. But the boozy, stoned atmosphere was immediately welcoming, and he found himself the recipient of a remarkable degree of friendliness from the people there.

It wasn't long, however, before he found he was getting both tired and over-intoxicated, and when one of the more intellectually-minded Music Matters people cornered him and finally embarked on a serious discussion about the politics of music, he became quite anxious about his inability to respond with any real coherence.

He found it hard to concentrate anyway, because the two girls he had stared at during the gig had come on to the party, and he couldn't take his eyes off them.

They were in many ways the life and soul of the occasion. They giggled, danced together even when no one else was dancing, sat on people's laps, put their arms round people, and kissed at least half the men at the party.

Tony watched them ravenously. It seemed to him that they were the epitome of the kind of girls he had always wanted but never had – loose, light-hearted, fun-loving, flagrantly sexy.

Once again he found himself puzzling over which one he fancied most, while simultaneously bemoaning the fact – he was quite sure it was a fact – that neither of them could possibly be the least bit interested in him. Although they behaved in similar ways, they were quite different in their appeal. The blonde was what blondes were traditionally supposed to be – curvy and big-breasted and bubbly and cuddly. The black-haired one, on the other hand, had a hint of fragility about her. Her slenderness and her big, dark eyes aroused protective feelings in him. Although her sexuality, like the blonde's, was overt, there was a greater mystery to it. He didn't know which of them his own sexuality was most suited to.

As he covertly ogled them from across the room, an uncalled-for thought entered his mind that made him feel more disturbed by them than ever. It was generally known – or at least generally believed – that girls who hung around the music scene were particularly willing to perform oral sex, and particularly good at it.

He was quite appalled to find himself thinking this, but the thought wouldn't go away. He was unable to prevent himself from glancing at the girls' mouths and wondering if indeed this was what they did.

At which point, Chas went over to the blonde girl and started doing a very publicly erotic dance with her, hunched over her in his fur coat (which he was still wearing despite the crush of people and the heat in the flat) and groping her bottom for all the world to see. Tony watched, sick with envy, wishing that he, too, was a shameless hedonist like Chas, and that he also had the gall to go up to people and grope them like that.

Not long after, Chas, having detached himself from the blonde, came over to him.

'How do you like our groupies?' he asked. It seemed, embarrassingly, that he had noticed where Tony's attention kept wandering.

Tony laughed uneasily.

'Your groupies, are they?'

'Yeah,' said Chas. 'They're the Music Matters groupies. You can't have a rock outfit without groupies, can you?'

It was almost as if Chas was serious. In spite of his own reaction to the girls, part of Tony's mind began to protest at this sexism. But he was forestalled from making any comment, first of all by noticing that Chas's crooked grin was now so wide that his face appeared to be almost split in half by it, and secondly by Chas's next remark, which was so astonishing that at first Tony didn't think he had really said what he seemed to have said.

'Would you like one for the night?' asked Chas.

'What?'

He gaped at Chas as if he had gone mad.

'Are you serious?' he managed to say at last.

Chas's demeanour became severe.

'I told you,' he said. 'When I said we'd give you a good time here, I meant it.'

Tony felt quite giddy. This could not possibly be happening. Yet evidently it was happening – and as this sank in, two voices inside his head began a high-speed debate with each other.

No, remonstrated one of them. You can't do such a thing. It's against everything you're supposed to believe in. Women's bodies are not to be disposed of in this way. You'd just be colluding with Chas's fantasies of being a pimp. The whole idea is sordid and grotesque beyond belief. Think what Sara would say, what all the people you respect would say. Think of your own respect for yourself!

Yes, insisted the other voice. This is exactly the kind of thing you've always dreamed about. Remember how you felt in the sixties, when everyone was getting stoned and being promiscuous, and you were kept back from all the fun by your loyalty to your wife – who, I might add, is probably being fucked silly by Joe this very minute. You've fantasized about this sort of thing happening for years. Well, now's your chance. Go for it, you'll always regret it if you don't.

The outcome was never really in doubt.

'Okay,' he said, and he gave Chas what he hoped was a cheerful, nonchalant grin.

Chas nodded and pursed his lips, as though to say: 'Sensible fellow, you made the right decision.' Then he turned and walked straight over to the two girls. The three of them held a conference, both girls glancing over towards Tony.

Tony waited, feeling intensely nervous.

Which girl was it going to be? And how in hell was the decision being made?

And how was he going to deal with it when it was made?

The skinny girl in black detached herself from the other two and came over to him.

'Hello,' she said.

Tony gave her a strained grin.

'Hello,' he said. '. . . My name's Tony. What's yours?'

'Anna,' she said.

'Uh-huh,' he said.

There was an awkward pause.

'. . . Do you fancy a dance?' he asked.

'Okay.'

They started dancing. Tony tried to get on top of the situation. Incredible as it seemed, this girl – this pretty girl who was now undulating in front of him – was going to go to bed with him.

That being the case, he decided it behoved him to come on a

bit, to show her that he was groovy and nice and it was all going to be jolly good fun.

Unfortunately, his problem with his dancing seemed to have returned. His limbs appeared to have developed a life of their own that was nothing to do with the record that was being played and still less to do with the movements of Anna's limbs. What's more, the smile he gave her every now and then was, he was certain, rigid and goofy.

She didn't seem to mind. While she didn't respond to his smile, she didn't look put out by it either. She seemed, in fact, to be thinking about something else.

Then she suddenly broke off dancing and went over to her blonde friend and started a whispered, giggling conversation with her. They both glanced across at someone else in the room. Tony decided that whatever Anna's motive for agreeing to sleep with him was, an interest in him as a person appeared to have very little to do with it.

His doubts about the situation began to resurface. Maybe this was all a bit of a mistake?

But the voice that had coaxed him into saying yes returned to reassure him. After all, it said, this was Chas's idea, not his. And so long as Anna wasn't being forced to do anything against her will . . .

Besides, he was intensely curious about what was going to happen. It was almost as if he had a responsibility to see the thing through. By doing so, he would be adding to the sum of human knowledge. He would certainly be adding to the sum of his own knowledge, anyway.

A sense of passivity came over him, as if he wasn't really a protagonist in what was going on. Things were happening to him that were being arranged by others. All he had to do was let them get on with it.

He glanced across the room at Anna's pert little face. How pretty she was! And what sexy clothes she wore!

This was the most exciting thing that had happened to him for ages. Why wasn't he more excited?

3.

The party ended at about 2 a.m., and he found her by his side again.

'Is it okay if I stay at your place?' he asked, still not quite believing what had been decided.

'Yeah, sure,' she said.

So they went out into the night and got into his car.

It had started to rain. They drove through dismal streets, the light from dull street-lamps reflecting back off wet pavements and roads, row after row of terraced, red-brick houses on either side, Anna directing him.

It was cold. He hunched himself up in his overcoat while he drove, and tried to find out more about Anna. She was at art college, she said, doing a course in graphic design. She helped out with the secretarial work at Music Matters, and designed some of the posters. It was she and her friend Suzy who had stuck up the posters for the concert round Manchester.

'Flyposting's good,' she said. 'It's fun. When the law stop us, we just flirt with them, and they let us go.'

She said this with relish, and Tony had a picture of Anna and Suzy as a team, larking about together and getting off on their solidarity with each other amongst the men.

'You're not really groupies, though, are you?' he asked.

'Yeah,' she said simply. 'Why not?'

He felt unable to probe her further about this, though he would have liked to, and when he asked her about her opinion of Music Matters, she just said:

'It's something to do, isn't it?'

At which point, the conversation rather dried up.

He started to feel uncomfortable. He thought to himself: she's not very bright. How did I get myself into this situation? This girl and I have absolutely nothing in common. This whole thing's absurd.

'Over on the left,' said Anna.

He drew up outside her house, and they went in through a wildly overgrown garden, stooping to avoid the wet branches of the trees that hung over the path.

Her room was bleak, cold and inadequately furnished. There were some rather weird psychedelic paintings and drawings on the walls – Anna's own work, she told him – but otherwise little apart from a pretty quilted bedspread that testified to her artistic bent.

Or was it simply that she was poor? The furniture and carpet looked as though they had been picked up from jumble-sales and second-hand shops, and instead of shelves for books there was merely a stack of orange boxes.

Anna lit a lamp by the bed and then draped a red cloth over it, so that it scarcely penetrated the dark. Then she lit the gas fire, and went into a corner of the room to make some coffee on the single gas-ring that apparently served as her kitchen.

'It'll have to be black,' she said. 'I've run out of milk.'

Her manner was most disconcerting. While they drank their coffee, he tried again to engage her in conversation, but without any success. She seemed indifferent to his attempts to create a friendly atmosphere between them. In fact – to put it simply – she seemed bored.

More and more he felt that it would be wrong to attempt to have sex with her after all. The desire he had felt for her earlier in the evening had vanished. He now felt that to try to fuck her would indeed be thoroughly exploitative. In any case he didn't feel like it, since she clearly didn't particularly like him.

He couldn't leave her, because he didn't have anywhere else to go. But they wouldn't fuck. He'd just give her a bit of friendship and a cuddle, and then go to sleep.

But when they had finished their coffee and smoked a joint and got into bed – Tony still wearing his shirt and pants as a protection against both Anna and the cold – she suddenly clung to him passionately, holding him tight and giving him violent kisses, her frail body shaking with emotion. There was no doubt at all about what she wanted.

'Are you sure we should?' he managed to say – but she just kept on pressing against him and shuddering, and her hand was already inside his pants, clutching at his prick, working it roughly up to an erection.

He decided that the matter was outside his control – or rather, that it would be ungentlemanly to refuse her, and that although he was far from sure he really wanted her, if she wanted him he would go along with it.

He shuffled out of his pants and then put his hand down between her legs and fingered her cunt. Her reaction was extraordinary. She sighed and panted and wriggled, pressing against his hand, rubbing herself roughly against him, not allowing a second's respite.

He still wasn't very much into what was happening, and his prick was only half hard. It occurred to him that maybe she would go down on him and suck him to turn him on more, as he had fantasized earlier in the evening. But she was already very wet, and everything about her behaviour indicated that she wanted him now. So he dutifully moved on top of her and, with a certain amount of difficulty, inserted himself inside her.

She immediately went wild. Strange guttural sounds came from her throat, and she clawed at his back and her body writhed and shook. He was impressed. This girl was seriously into sex! Perhaps he was going to have a good time after all?

But when he pushed further into her, it was as if she was retreating from him, twisting away. He pushed again, and again she retreated, making a sound that was very much like a laugh.

Was this some kind of teasing? he wondered. Something was going on that he didn't quite understand. But Anna was still heaving and thrashing about under him, so he pushed into her again.

She suddenly grabbed a handful of his hair, and pulled it hard.

'Ow!' he said, and froze.

But then she pushed against him again, working her sinewy body at him and making little, desperate, demanding noises, telling him to go on.

So he did, and again she retreated, writhing, twisting about, clawing at him, biting his shoulder. And he suddenly realized what was happening: she was *fighting* him.

She wanted him to be violent with her, and she wanted to be violent back . . .

For as long as he could he went along with it. As soon as she realized that he had understood what was going on, she laughed again, and attacked him more vigorously than ever. He tried to pin her down, to hold her skinny arms so that she couldn't scratch him, and she laughed her weird laugh and panted and fought herself free and started to claw at him and beat him again. Her strength was astonishing. When she grabbed a handful of his flesh and squeezed it, she really hurt him. And when she bit him it was excruciating.

The outcome of the battle was never decided. His prick, which had briefly taken an interest in the proceedings, wilted rapidly as soon as the situation became one which he was dealing with exclusively with his intellect. And once it slipped out of her, she immediately subsided, all her aggression gone. She took his prick in her hand and tried to press it into her again, but to no avail. He wondered if now she would after all try to suck him to make him hard again, but the idea no longer appealed to him. Without any doubt at all, she would bite it off.

He folded her in his arms and held her tight, and this time there was no resistance. She let him stroke her head and be tender with her.

'I think I'm too drunk to carry on,' he said.

She didn't say anything, just turned round so that her back was to him, and prepared to go to sleep. He wrapped himself round her, for warmth and for his comfort and hers, and gradually his panting and the beating of his heart calmed down, and the northern darkness pressed in on him.

They slept till late. When they finally got up, Anna appeared even more listless and abstracted than she had the night before. But she evidently bore him no animosity, and they chatted vaguely and casually as if their bout in bed had never happened.

He had another cup of black coffee, and then drove her into town to see a friend.

'Bye,' she said, when she parted from him, and he watched her walk away, a pretty girl in an old fur coat like Chas's, her skinny legs still perched on high-heeled shoes – a girl that, seeing her for the first time on the streets, he might have followed with his eyes and thought: I wonder what she's like?

Then he drove off to meet the Music Matters people again. They were having a meeting during the afternoon, and he was supposed to attend and take notes.

When he found the house and went in, they were grouped together in the kitchen, drinking coffee.

'So she didn't break your arm, then,' said Chas nonchalantly, and one of the others laughed.

Tony was shocked. Had the whole business been some kind of warped practical joke?

But the Music Matters people were as cheerfully friendly to him as before, and they went on to talk about Anna with fondness rather than scorn. Tony decided that the situation was simply beyond his understanding, and just smiled back at them and tried to keep his cool.

He didn't leave the meeting until it was already getting dark.

Driving back to London, a feeling of bleakness and emptiness that had lurked with him all day finally took over. He felt cold and weary and used – not used by Anna, nor by the others, but by himself. He felt as if he had done himself some thoughtless, unnecessary damage.

d.i.y.

mary scott

It was always the same the night Helen returned from holiday. She couldn't sleep.

She'd tried everything: milky drinks, a warm bath, interesting books, dull books, a small glass of wine, a large one of whisky. If she switched on the light and read, would that lull her brain? Or stimulate it? Tonight she opted for staying stock still and concentrating on an imaginary square of black velvet: which was her latest technique.

It didn't work. It never failed to amaze her how, once she was alone in bed, her unconscious could take charge and present her with images she'd really rather forget. Tonight it came up with Pete.

She could have been dwelling on Mario's charms. While nothing, she reflected, beat good sex for curing insomnia, second best was reliving good sex recently enjoyed. So her holidays sometimes brought weeks on end of deep, uninterrupted slumber. Though not on the first night.

She put it down to the change in lifestyle: she didn't have sex at home.

What had reminded her of Pete? Someone on the plane? At Gatwick? No, it was the luscious Mario himself. He couldn't accept the holiday for what it was, started insisting they meet again, wanted her address, said he was in London quite often on business. For one, the mention of business spoiled her pleasure; she wanted to remember him lying half-naked and tanned on a hot beach, not trussed up in a three-piece suit. For two, she couldn't have her foreign partners-in-sex turning up and intruding on her life; what would people think of a succession of Spaniards, Germans, Frenchmen? Of course she'd keep them well away from the office; but still, word would be bound to get about. So she gave Mario a false address. But when they said goodbye he was still frantically scribbling down his own address and going on about how he'd look her up, they should keep in touch, at least be friends. As if she would have sex with a friend!

She did that with Pete.

They were at university together, she and Pete, were best mates. Until they got pissed and ended up in bed.

This was a horrible thing to recall. She remembered how, on penetration, she sobered up and saw Pete pumping up and down, saw his face, close up, all its familiar, lively intelligence wiped away by the fatuous emptiness of lust. Afterwards they hardly spoke to each other again.

She glared up at the dark ceiling. Damn Mario for stirring up old memories. Why couldn't he accept that the best sex was anonymous? Still, it was only four months ago that she'd spent that glorious no-strings week in Lanzarote with Kurt; she decided to concentrate on remembering him. She fell asleep.

Monday morning. Helen's first consultation was with Louise Saunders. According to her file she wanted to discuss options for topping up her allowable expenditure: for tax purposes.

But first, 'How was the holiday?' Louise asked.

'Wonderful. I exhausted myself doing absolutely nothing,' lied Helen, 'Except for flopping around on the beach and eating superb meals. It was cheap too. Would be even cheaper if they didn't slap on a single room supplement.'

'You mean you went on your own?'

She nodded. 'Always do. Makes it an adventure. And you see so much more than if you're with a crowd.'

'I wish I had your nerve. I'm for ever holidaying with people I *think* are friends. Who end up, after a couple of weeks of living together, as anything but.'

'You should try going solo.'

After Louise left, Luke stuck his head round the door. 'Spare a moment?'

'Sure. Even a coffee if you want one.'

He asked about the trip. She gave him the expurgated version.

'Sounds great.'

Helen stifled a small yawn. 'Tiring though. The flight back was delayed,' she lied again.

He took his coffee and propped himself on the edge of her desk. 'The other reason I popped in . . That awkward corner you mentioned. In your hallway. Have you found something for it yet?'

'Nope. Any suggestions?'

'New place just opened in Camden Passage. Saw some promising-looking deco stuff in the window.'

She wrinkled her nose.

'Added to which,' he went on, 'it might wean you off that bakelite junk you were waxing lyrical about.'

'Fifties pieces have increased in value.' She settled her own cup on her desk, beside her diary, then added, 'Oh Lord, look. Jane's booked me to see Deborah at 11.30 and I haven't even mugged up on her file. Sorry Luke, I'll have to catch you later.'

That weekend, though, she did try the place he'd suggested; she didn't find a thing. But while she was out and about she might as well go further afield. She drove around north London, eyes peeled for likely places. Eventually she fetched up, still empty-handed, in Walthamstow. And look, *there* was a furniture shop, well, more a junk shop really; but it could be worth a glance. She pulled over and parked.

She opened the shop door with care (the glass panel was cracked), stepped inside; and came face to face with the most stunning man. None of her foreign lovers could even hope to compete. She gazed at him. God, he must spend hours on a sunbed. And at the gym. Hang on there, what was he saying? Oh, he was asking whether she had anything particular in mind. She shook her head, then nodded it and launched, swiftly, into what she wanted in the way of furniture. He nodded too, then unearthed a sort of ghastly modern what-not made, so far as she could tell, of plywood. He had to move a great heap of other junk to get at it, which gave her the opportunity to watch biceps and pecs in action.

A pity she hadn't come across him somewhere *abroad*, she mourned. Which is when it occurred to her. Why should she have to stick to foreigners? London was a big place and this guy was a complete stranger; not in a million years would he know anyone she did. Besides she still wasn't sleeping all that well, on account of the nasty taste Mario had left.

She made up her mind. Tactics next. Would her best bet be to buy the thing and have him deliver it? But if she did she'd be stuck with the monstrosity; otherwise he'd notice it wasn't there every time he came round to her flat.

'Yes?' she realized he was asking. 'Or no?'

She shook her head again. 'But now you know what I want . . .?'

'I'll keep an eye out.'

She was used to working fairly fast: her holidays were rarely longer than a week. So two return trips to the shop and she had an assignation fixed up. Come the next weekend the stunning-looking man was sitting beside her on her rather nice Edwardian chaise.

It turned out that she'd struck lucky. Because – although

her new lover could hardly string two words together – he had a brilliant imagination where sex was concerned.

Over the next few weeks he came up with the most unusual uses for a whole variety of household objects. None of your ready-made sex toys for him; he improvised. With scraps of slippery, cool leather; with all the belts in her wardrobe; with a couple of chunky, gold bracelets; a hairband; a silk scarf each; and the entire contents of the rather nice crystal dish in which she kept her fresh fruit. Some evenings he even raided the fridge hungrily for a bag of carrots or a cool, green cucumber.

On second thoughts, she reflected, one night as she lay in bed after he'd left, maybe he wasn't imaginative, just strapped for cash and had to use whatever came to hand. What did she care? She hadn't slept so well in years.

Everyone at work noticed her extra energy. Luke said she was in fine fettle. *She* said had he seen *Poirot* the previous night, seeing as he was so keen on thirties decor? He said was she watching *Lipstick on Your Collar* seeing she was so set on the fifties? Turned out they'd both been watching both. At which point Helen turfed him out; she had another appointment with Louise.

'You look so *well* these days,' Louise declared the moment she was seated. 'All those holidays certainly pay off.'

'But I've only had two this year. My usual quota's three.'

'And every one on your own?' Helen nodded. Louise shook her head at her boldness.

This time she wanted advice on putting her growing savings to work. She specified ethical investments only; Helen explained she didn't recommend anything but. The phone rang. 'Won't keep you a moment.' She picked it up.

'Helen Haliwell,' she told the mouthpiece. For a moment there was no reply. She repeated her name. Then her lover began to talk. Dirty. Helen felt her face grow hot. This must be his latest bright idea, she realized. And an utterly appalling one. Suppose Louise could hear? Helen shot a quick look at her, but she sat unmoved. At the other end of the line Helen's lover was painting a picture – not a very articulate one but she certainly got the gist – of how the white flesh of her buttocks would look criss-crossed with thin black leather thongs. 'Sandra,' she told him, 'I'm in conference. Could we discuss these details later?' And dumped the receiver on its rest. Was she blushing? She couldn't have been: as Louise was waiting, calmly, for her to continue.

On Saturday Helen told her lover in no uncertain terms what she thought of him. She told him he must never, *ever* phone her at work. He grinned at her vehemence and reminded her of several other activities she hadn't taken to straight off. Then he started moving mirrors about so they could see themselves having sex from every angle. They did. It was as good as ever; so was her night's rest.

Sunday morning she rose early, went to Brick Lane. She got a great kick out of haggling, energetically, over a nicely-proportioned reproduction deco lamp and came away only ten pounds lighter and with a feeling of considerable triumph. Luke would approve of this purchase too.

Monday, in the office, she was describing it to him when the phone rang.

She picked it up and a stream of filth poured into her ear.

She didn't dare look at Luke. She felt sure he couldn't hear, Louise hadn't. But this was beyond a joke. It was worse than fifty Marios turning up on the office doorstep. She slammed down the phone.

Luke raised an eyebrow. 'Problems?'

She assured him not. 'But I must get on.'

'Fair enough. Are you coming to the drinks do on Friday?'

She nodded.

Immediately after work she phoned her lover and ditched him. He said why and couldn't they keep in touch? She said no and you know why. He said he wouldn't phone again, not like that. She said it was too late. He said hadn't it all been fun? She said there was no point in going over old ground and he hadn't even found her a decent piece of furniture. He said why didn't she drop into the shop; he had something he was sure she'd like. She said no again. And then, just like Mario, he said couldn't they at least be friends? What on earth would she want to be friends with him for? She put down the phone thanking God she was out of that; and slept surprisingly well.

At the drinks do Luke made a bee-line for her; she'd thought he might, they hadn't had much opportunity for a proper chat recently. They talked furniture of course, then television, then cinema. They progressed to paintings and discovered a shared passion for Carpaccio. They talked and talked.

Of course she should have known where they were heading. But she hadn't done things this way for so very, very long. She was used to making all the running with a man who either didn't speak her language or, in the case of her ex-lover, wasn't fluent in his own. So when Luke leant forward and touched her arm, quite lightly, she almost recoiled with shock. He retracted his hand and rubbed his chin. 'I've been going, for ages, to suggest we team up one weekend and go to Brick Lane together. But you're always so busy. And last time your damn phone rang at the crucial moment.'

Jane butted in, a bottle of wine in either hand. 'Helen,' she said. She topped up their glasses. 'You know when you were in the loo getting ready for this evening?'

'Yes.'

'I took two calls in your office. Whoever it was hung up when I spoke. Must be a nuisance caller.' Helen could feel herself growing hot. 'Was that an anonymous call you had the other day?' asked Luke. 'If so you should notify BT.'

'No,' she told him. 'They were probably wrong numbers,'

she told Jane, then abandoned the pair of them. She homed in, on the opposite side of the room, on Louise.

'Lovely party,' said Louise, 'and timed exactly right for me.'

Out of the corner of her eye Helen could see Luke looking, puzzled, in her direction. She didn't look back. Louise was telling her that she'd finally decided to take a leaf out of her, Helen's, book. She was off – in a few days' time – for two weeks in the sunny Seychelles.

'God, that's what I could do with,' said Helen.

'I'm not quite as bold as you yet,' Louise rattled on. 'Though I'm not going with so-called friends this time. I *am* going under the auspices of a wonderful women-only travel group I've found. Great idea, isn't it? I can be on my own when I want, but there's always someone to talk to. Without any hassle. I can't imagine why I didn't think of it before.'

Helen couldn't either. The way she felt it sounded like an answer to a prayer. A week off. With no men. No ex-lover phoning. No embarrassing approaches from Luke. No sense of everything being just a little too close for comfort.

She didn't sleep a wink that night.

Saturday she rang the number Louise had given her. She was determined to go the following week so she had to take pot luck. They offered her Venice. Supposed to be a city for lovers to visit, wasn't it? she thought as she replaced the receiver. But what the hell.

All week she jumped whenever the phone went. She unplugged it several minutes before each client was due. Thankfully, Luke didn't drop in even once. Her ex-lover, though, called several times. He wasn't talking dirty now, simply going on and on about why couldn't they get together. Twice, when Helen was at lunch or in the loo, Jane took the calls. On those occasions he hung up.

At home Helen kept the answerphone switched on. Her nights were restless; but she had seven whole days of relaxation to look forward to: in pleasant, undemanding, uncomplicated company. And surely her ex-lover would give up after a week?

She was soon proved right about Venice being a city for lovers to visit. That's what all the other women on the plane were. It had hardly taken off before the two across the aisle were drinking champagne out of each other's plastic glasses, laughing and leaning all over each other to look out of the window. Behind Helen were several more pairs of women: all wrapped up in each other, all as happy as larks. The plane vibrated with the same buzz of sexuality as the one which transported the 18–30s group with whom she'd visited Ibiza in her early travelling days.

She looked at the empty seat beside her, ate her airline meal, drank some wine, then gazed gloomily down upon the peaks of the Alps. They were spectacular, like row upon row of slabs of dark, rich fruit cake, with a thick white icing of crusty snow. All around her women were oohing and aahing, enjoying the scenery in each other's company. She sat silent.

And that just about set the tone for the trip. They arrived at Venice airport. She kept herself to herself. The party piled into a motor boat. It set off across the lagoon. Normally she'd have been eyeing a likely foreigner. Failing that she'd have struck up a conversation with a middle-aged couple, say. She'd have found *someone* with whom to share that first, magical sight of the city, its buildings looming black through the mist, yellow light glancing on the silky water. As it was she didn't speak to anyone, she was afraid she might be misinterpreted, how she didn't know.

They were all staying at the same hotel, just off the Piazza San Marco, couldn't ask for a better location. But while everyone else clattered joyously into the foyer, eyes alight, talking nineteen to the dozen, Helen trailed behind like the one schoolgirl in the entire class who hasn't managed to find a best friend.

But though the company was not as she'd imagined, the city far exceeded expectation. She explored the island from end to end, stepping up and over the little grey bridges, peering into flagged, sunny courtyards, strolling down narrow, cool, brown-walled alleys. Venice was crowded, but she nosed out its quietest quarters, the smaller, humbler buildings to the south-west with sluggish channels slapping at their brick-work, lines of washing drooping overhead; and the leafier, wider walkways to the north. Sometimes she paused and gazed; at a vista of open water, a magnificent palace or a tiny shrine set in a crumbling wall and adorned with a posy of fresh flowers. She took herself off to the Accademia and lingered for hours over the Carpaccios that Luke and she both liked. At night she watched the moon preside over the choppy black waters of the Giudecca canal and the angular skyline of the island beyond. And she realized that she had never been so alone in her life. On her usual holidays she quickly found a lover. At home she had work and antique hunting to keep her occupied. Here she was utterly by herself, knew no one, no one knew her; and she loved it.

Most evenings she was starving after all her exercise. She returned to the hotel, showered and set off again. She went from restaurant to restaurant, teasing her appetite almost beyond endurance as she inspected the menus outside and inhaled the rich scents of garlic, aubergine, tomatoes and fresh fish wafting from within. When her stomach could stand no more, she ate. When she had eaten, she walked back to the Piazza and fell, exhausted, into bed.

She even slept well on her first night home.

Back at work Jane greeted her eagerly. 'You should have said before what the problem was,' she declared. 'With those phone calls, I mean.'

So Helen's ex-lover had found his tongue after all.

Jane hurried on. 'First he didn't say a word. Then, after he must have called at least ten times, he suddenly piped up. I was sure he wasn't *bona fide*. I figured he probably latched on to you, made a pest of himself during that week you spent in Marbella. After all, if you wanted to see him you'd have given him your home number, not left him to track you down at work. So I was pretty cagey about when you were scheduled to return. Anyway he'll be back in Spain by now. I took his address, just in case.' She handed Helen a piece of paper. And,' she added with an air of satisfaction, 'he hasn't called a single time since.'

Helen thanked her, looked down at Mario's address and threw the paper away.

That weekend she didn't shop around for something for the awkward corner in her hall. Instead she borrowed, from the library, a couple of books on DIY and one on Italian architecture. Then she went to Soho and bought a vibrator. She must remember to pack it on her next trip – where? In the evening she watched a video of *Don't Look Now* and recalled, fondly, the Bridge of Sighs and the waterbuses chugging along the Grand Canal between the elaborate façades of grey, yellow, red, blue palaces. She slept like a log.

fade to black

ian breakwell

June 3rd

On the wall opposite the bed was a full length mirror framed with gilt. He lay between her legs, licking her. She trembled. He swivelled and plunged his face between her thighs, gripping her buttocks with his hands. Her tongue flicked round his groin as she strained to reach his prick. Her little finger worked its way inside him. He swung round, lifted up her legs and slid his prick into her. She gasped. He groaned. Her hands clutched his shoulderblades. His tongue was in her ear. She came. He pulled out. She turned over on to her hands and knees. He slid into her again. He licked the fingers of her right hand so that she could rub herself at the same time. She pushed her face into the pillow. He gripped her hips. The bed creaked. The quilt had fallen on to the floor. In the mirror he could see her buttocks pressed against him. She came again. He withdrew and she rolled over. She sucked his prick, holding his balls in her hand. She moved to the edge of the bed, her feet on the floor. He stood between her legs. She lifted her feet until her knees were against her chest. He covered his prick with Vaseline and pushed it up her arse. Her mouth opened wide, then she pulled him down towards her. Her hand went down to her crotch. She said: 'Oh, I'm coming again.' He said: 'Go on then.' They came together, jerking like mario-nettes. Hard core of despair fending off the last goodbyes. She said: 'We could never just be friends. You know if you walk through that door it's the last time you'll ever see me.'

June 9th

He cooked a meal. They had steak, potatoes, salad and a bottle of wine. He washed the pots and she poured the coffee. After the coffee they stood in the middle of the room clutching each other. He unbuttoned her blouse. She unzipped his trousers. He put his hand up her skirt and pulled her tights down below her buttocks, then slipped his hand inside her pants. She knelt on the carpet and sucked him. His fingernails scraped her scalp. He took the coffee cups off the dinner table. She removed the cruet while holding his prick with her other hand. He helped her up on to the table. She lay on her back with her buttocks on the edge, her skirt above her waist. He pulled off her shoes, tights and pants. Her legs were bent upwards, suspended in mid-air. He stood with his trousers round his ankles, spread her legs and pushed it in. They both breathed 'Aaah' at the same time. On the wooden shelf behind her was a jar of Hortex Pickled Onions, a bottle of Lea & Perrins Worcester Sauce, a jar of Gales Pure Country Honey, three tins of Heinz Oven Baked Beans, and a jar of Nescafé Blend 37 Freeze Dried Instant Coffee. He slid in and out of her as she gripped the edge of the table with her hands. On the second shelf was a jar of Crosse & Blackwell Branston Pickle, a packet of Lyons Orange Label Tea, two tins of Heinz Tomato Soup and a box of Weetabix Whole Wheat Cereal Standard Size. Outside the window, beyond the black silhouettes of the plane trees, the lights shone brightly in the house opposite. 'They can see us,' she said. 'I don't care,' he said. And a tin of Napoli Peeled Plum Tomatoes, a jar of Colmans Mustard, a packet of Batchelors Dried Peas. Her face turned red, her eyes closed. He rested, still inside her, then withdrew and rubbed the tip of his prick backwards and forwards against her clitoris, then pushed hard into her. She lifted her buttocks to meet him. On the third shelf was a packet of Sainsburys Bread Sauce Mix, a bottle of Sarsons Malt Vinegar, a jar of Frank Coopers Mint Sauce, a tin of Lyons Original Blend Pure Ground Coffee, a packet of Bisto Gravy Mix and a bottle of H.P. Sauce. His eyes scanned the ingredients on the sauce bottle label: vinegar, tomatoes, dates, molasses, sugar, salt, rye, flour, edible starch, onions, tamarinds, spices, soy sauce, caramel, garlic, mustard, flavouring. Serve with hot meats, especially sausages, bacon, hamburgers, chops and cold meats. Delicious with cheese, fried eggs, fish and chips. Adds flavour to stews and casseroles. He thrust in and out of her faster now. He leaned forward as she clenched her teeth. Next to her left ear on the table top was a smear of mustard. They came together, gasping and shuddering. He pulled out, walked to the sink and brought back a paper tissue roll. She sat on the edge of the table and wiped herself. He said: 'Would you like another cup of coffee?' She said: 'Yes, please.' He put the coffee back on the stove. They sat at opposite ends of the table, drank their coffee and smoked cigarettes. When they had stubbed out their cigarettes she said: 'It's as if it never happened.' He said: 'Let's go out for a drink.'

June 14th

She lay back on the bed, naked except for the broad belt with the silver clasp around her waist. He scooped moisturising cream out of the jar. He lifted her left foot, holding the heel in the palm of his hand. He rubbed the cream into the instep, sole and ankle, and in between each toe. Then the other foot. Then both feet together until they were oily and smooth, sliding backwards and forwards in his hands as little worms of cream

squeezed out between his fingers. 'Nice?' he said. 'Mmmm.'
Her eyes closed and she smiled. His thumb was deep inside her
cunt. His little finger, greased with cream, was up her arse. His
left hand still massaged her right foot. Her right hand reached
out towards his mouth. He licked her fingertips. She rubbed
her clitoris as his tongue flicked between her circling fingers.
His hands stretched up to her breasts, pinching the erect
nipples. She held him by the hair and gripped his head with her
thighs. He held her down as she shuddered.

June 29th

This time last year: we walked along the coastal path and
stood hip to hip on the cliff top above the sea. Cormorants
skimmed over the waves. A seal was rolling among the rocks
below. The sun shone down from a blue sky. We hugged each
other, laughing, our noses in each other's hair, then lay down
naked in the warm grass.

Today: he knocked three times. She opened the door with a
wry smile, holding a Siamese kitten in her left hand. After tea
and cigarettes they stood in front of the mirror. He lifted her
skirt. She unbuttoned his flies and pulled out his prick, then
leaned forward and sucked him, his fingers still inside her. She
squatted by the mirror and put her diaphragm in. The kitten
stood unsteadily on the carpet, gazing up at them and mewing.
He stood on the other side of the mirror, his prick sticking out
of his pin-stripe suit. She pulled his trousers down. He sat on
the chair and she straddled him, her arms round his neck as
she eased down on to his prick. He grasped her buttocks. She
worked up and down and side to side. He pulled her sweater
up above her breasts and sucked her nipples. She said: 'I'm
going to come, I'm going to come.' He said: 'Go on, go on.'
Her fingers dug into his back. She was shouting. Then she
stopped and said: 'I thought you were going to come with me?

Why didn't you?' He said: 'I don't know, I thought I would but I didn't.' She said: 'I see.' Her face set. Her lips pressed tightly together and she turned to one side. He said: 'Shall we carry on?' She said: 'If you like.'

July 1st

This time last year: in the evening sunshine we sat drinking gin and tonics on the terrace of the cottage surrounded by hedges of wild fuchsia. On the side of the hill the black mare and its foal walked slowly across the field. Rooks circled over the trees on the brow of the hill. In the bay far below the waves rolled silently in to the deserted beach. We kissed again and again. With our arms round each other we went inside and up the stairs, still kissing, then lay on the bed and rubbed oil all over each other's suntanned bodies, then made love, and at the end we shouted so loud together that we burst out laughing afterwards, and she said: 'They must have heard us in the village.' Then we fell asleep in each other's arms.

Today: they went to her flat and ate a meal. Silence settled on them like a blanket. Three hours later he said: 'I think I'll go.' He put on his jacket and walked down the corridor to the door. She ran out of the room and swung him round by the shoulder. She punched him in the mouth, on the nose, the side of the head and in the eyes. She kicked him in the groin, calling him a swine, a bastard, an unfeeling rat. The kitten cowered behind a chair, its ears flat against its head. He recovered his composure. They went out to the pub and drank against the clock, then walked back to the flat. They took off their clothes, she lay back on the bed and opened her legs. He knelt between her thighs and licked her, pressing his left hand on her pubic bone, two fingers pushed deep in her cunt, his thumb pressed against her arse. She came, writhing on the bed, her flesh moving in ripples up her stomach as the spasms shook her. He lay flat on his back with her reversed above him. Her breasts were squashed against his stomach. She held his balls and sucked him frantically. He thrust his tongue between the pink lips as she ground her cunt against his face. She swallowed and sat up, sperm running down from the corner of her mouth. They stared at each other blankly. She put the light out and they lay back to back. It was a night of fitful sleep. In the morning there was nothing to say. She made coffee and went off to work. He lay in bed staring at the wall. The kitten settled on his head, purring loudly.

July 3rd

It was a hot and airless night. She lay naked on her stomach on the bed. He sat astride her, his balls pressing against the cleft between her buttocks, his prick sticking out in front of him. With the fingernails of both hands he scratched her shoulder-blades, the back of her ribcage and up and down her spine from the nape of her neck to the small of her back. He moved down the bed and knelt astride her legs, lightly scratching her buttocks and the backs of her thighs and calves. Taking hold of her ankles he parted her legs. He leaned forward and pressed his lips between her buttocks, pushing the tip of his tongue into her arsehole which at first constricted and then opened as she raised herself with her elbows. She rolled over and lifted her knees. He licked her, two fingers of his right hand deep inside her, the base of his hand pressed hard against the ridge between her cunt and arse. His left hand was cupped underneath her, and she lifted her buttocks to meet his movements as he moved his tongue around her clitoris, then licked and fingered her very fast until she came with convulsive heaves, pressing her pubic bone hard against his upper lip. He licked her slowly for a time as she lazily rubbed herself, then she moved down the bed, impaled him on her little finger and began to suck him. He locked his legs around her neck and they rolled from side to side with his prick in her mouth to the root. The clock on the bedside table said 1.10 a.m. His concentration drifted. He remembered this time last summer when they wandered together through the lanes leading down to the sea and she pointed out to him all the different wild flowers which filled the hedgerows and the fields, naming each in turn as he listened enraptured: Pennywort, Dropwort, Vetch, Scabious, Fuchsia, Honeysuckle, Ragwort, Bedstraw, Groundsel, Spear Thistle, Sheeps Bit, Cowslip, Bellflowers, Speedwell, Angelica, Hedge Parsley, Sea Holly, Yellow Loosestrife, Summer Gorse, Fringed Rock Cress, Sea Milkwort, Musk Mallow, Scarlet Pimpernel, Evening Primrose and Forget Me Nots. His prick went limp in her mouth. She took it out, frowned at him and said: 'What's the matter?' 'Nothing,' he said. She sighed and lay down with her back to him. He pulled the bedclothes over them and switched off the light. Numb despair froze him rigid. Sleep would not come. Every time he closed his eyes he saw a smooth grey rectangle, its surface covered with a dull sheen. A hundred times he closed his eyes and a hundred times the dreadful grey form re-appeared. No monsters. No demons. No stuff that dreams are made of. Just the lifeless monochrome of the nightmare.

In the morning it felt as if there was an iron band around his neck. Teeth clamped tight. Hands clenched into fists. Every muscle in his body ached. As if he had been beaten with telephone directories. Veins injected with plastic wood. He lay like a fish on a slab. She stood at the foot of the bed, tapped him on the ankle and said: 'I have to leave in half an hour, you must get up.' He turned his head. An inch away were the eyes of the cat. The cat looked into his dead fish eyes and backed away, jumped off the bed and slunk out of the room.

July 29th

He embraced her. She embraced him. He held her tight. She turned her head to one side, flicked her gas lighter and lit a cigarette. His arms fell to his sides. She leaned over the table and inspected the dried-up flowers of the plant on the window ledge. She touched each of the dead blooms in turn with her fingertips, leaning further forward with her pelvis pressed against the edge of the table. Standing behind her he lifted her skirt and pulled down her pants. He knelt on the linoleum and kissed her buttocks as she pruned the plant with a pair of scissors. She said: 'Shall we go to the pub?' He said: 'Sure.'

In the bar they sat at the corner table underneath the clock. An hour passed in silence. They responded politely when someone sat down nearby, borrowed a match, hung their coats on the hook behind them, or the barmaid changed the ashtray. After an hour it was closing time. She pulled on her jacket, glanced towards him and said brightly: 'O.K?' He gathered up his cigarettes and matches and said decisively: 'O.K.' They walked back to the car three feet apart. He stared ahead through the windscreen and said: 'Maybe we need to get away. A holiday. Back to where we've been happy.'

August 8th

On the bedside table is a vase containing a bouquet of honeysuckle, fuchsia and summer gorse. The rain beats down on the skylight above the bed on which he is lying naked on his back. His arms are stretched out on either side, his wrists tied tightly with two nylon stockings to the iron bedposts at the top of the bed. His legs are open, stretched out, each ankle tied to the bedposts at the bottom of the bed. He is gagged by means of a piece of cloth with several turns between the teeth. She is standing on the far side of the bedroom, smiling. She stubs out her cigarette in the ashtray on the bedside table, removes her shoes, stockings and pants, and climbs on to the bed. She kneels astride, facing him. She unfastens her belt and unbuttons her dress down the side, then slowly pulls it over her head. She unhooks her bra and drops it on to the floor beside the bed, on top of the dress and shoes. She unbraids her long hair and trails it across his body and face. Then, starting at his toes, she licks him with slow tongue strokes, over his insteps, ankles and calves, up his thighs, across his belly and chest, along each arm, into each palm, around his neck, beneath his chin and round each eye. Next, holding him by his hair, she rubs his face against her armpits and breasts. Then she locks her legs round his neck, presses her crotch against his face, and parting the labia with her fingers she pushes against his nose and upper lip. She places one hand over his eyes and with the other she traces a path with her fingernails down his chest and belly and around his groin, then lightly strokes his prick with her thumb and forefinger. Then she sits on his chest, her buttocks against his chin, and holding the base of his prick with her left hand she masturbates him with her right, alternating a slow, languid rhythm with quick, nervous strokes. Now she turns and kneels between his thighs. As she holds his balls with her right hand she licks him along the length of his prick from the base to the tip, then takes him into her mouth and begins to suck, at first slowly, then faster and faster, her nipples brushing against the hairs on the insides of his thighs. Sweat breaks out on his forehead as he writhes helplessly. His eyes shut tight. His teeth bite into the gag. His fingernails dig into his palms. Spasms run through him from head to toe. He thrashes from side to side, then slowly subsides. She straightens up and wipes her mouth with the back of her hand. She smiles. His breathing returns to normal. His eyes begin to close.

When he awoke she was no longer in the room. The rain had stopped. A breeze stirred the closed curtains. The sun shone brightly through the skylight on to his face.

The sweat had dried on his body. He shivered.

His movements had tightened the knots in the stockings which secured his hands and feet. He flexed his fingers and toes and shifted position as best he could, to try to ease the numbness in his limbs. He listened carefully. There was no sound from downstairs.

A seagull circled high above the skylight, drifting in the windcurrents.

The sky was blue and there were no clouds during the afternoon.

The sun began to set. The sky through the skylight was red.

By dusk the wind had dropped. He could hear the sound of the waves breaking against the foot of the cliffs below the cottage, and the raucous calls of the rooks coming home to roost in the woods on the hillside. In the distance the cries of the curlews in the estuary.

The light began to fade. A moth fluttered against the skylight then settled on his face.

A spider spun a web between the bedpost and the wall.

It became dark.

morning always comes

matt cohen

It all began with her skin. If not for her skin . . . But before Carolyn's skin there was Sarah.

Hugh went to bed with Sarah after two years of nervous courtship that vacillated between friendship and flirtation. 'Let's do it, just to prove we can,' Sarah finally said. Hugh would never have made such a proposition, which didn't mean he didn't want to. Sarah was dark, thin, smart and Hugh admired everything about her from the books she read and the music she could identify over the radio to the way she laughed without worrying about her teeth and her generous habit of cooking exquisite meals to which she regularly invited him. On these occasions they drank French red wine, supplied by Hugh, and had joke-telling contests. As they were pulling the sheet over their heads, Sarah said, 'Don't hurt me.'

'Don't worry,' replied Hugh. He was so nervous he was afraid he would be unable to inflict pleasure, let alone pain. Later Sarah told Hugh his peculiar response was what made her trust him, a burden Hugh carried faithfully while Sarah, it turned out, focused elsewhere.

When Hugh left Sarah and came back to Toronto from Paris, he installed himself in the third floor apartment of a large downtown brick house. It had attractions. The landlord was an old friend from other eras. Also, the apartment was reachable not only from the front entrance, which led past the landlord's ground floor apartment, but via a fire escape in the back. Hugh liked the idea of being able to come and go unobserved, even when he had no destinations in mind.

The apartment was furnished with a few Salvation Army basics – two frayed red armchairs, a paint-covered kitchen table, a rug that had seen better days. Details were still missing.

One day in a hardware store near his house, he saw a cappuccino coffee maker, complete with little nozzles for spraying hot milk. Hugh was not a cappuccino drinker, but due to his sparse furniture and all the sad events that had driven him from Sarah in Paris to a threadbare existence in Toronto, he wanted something fancy. The coffee maker resembled a large three-dimensional coat of arms in brass and stainless steel. Coincidentally, Hugh was carrying an empty tennis bag. It belonged to his landlord friend. Hugh was not a tennis player; the bag functioned as a giant briefcase in which Hugh carried losing entries to the annual Canadian Broadcasting Corporation memoirs contest for which he was one of the judges. Having returned a few dozen losers to the Corporation headquarters, Hugh was on his way home, empty-bagged, and had stopped at the hardware store thinking to buy a straw mat upon which to wipe his feet come the inevitable rainy day.

Without thinking he hoisted the coffee maker into his bag. It was heavy and the first thing Hugh realized was that it was important to leave the store with his shoulders parallel. Proud of his instant criminal savvy, Hugh started walking. That was when he saw Carolyn.

If not for her skin he would have kept on walking, out the store and onto the street. Life would have been a cup of cappuccino coffee. But, perhaps because there are no free cups of coffee, he paused, undecided, and then he couldn't stop staring. Her skin was smooth with an unplaceable golden cast. He thought it must be the light.

She was sitting at the cash register and when she looked up at him, the light broke apart the colour of her eyes. 'Can I help you?' As he was asking himself if he found her skin attractive or just unusual, his tennis bag split open.

A depressing scene took place in the back office of the store. The participants were Hugh, a somewhat bemused policeman who'd been hauled in from giving parking tickets, and the gold-skinned woman – who was also the owner. She was very tense, chestnut-haired, mid-thirties. She wanted Hugh behind bars. She didn't seem the type to own a hardware store and that was the problem. The previous owner, her father, had recently died. The store, due to the recession, was unsaleable. The woman had left a perfectly good job teaching remedial reading in the Northwest Territories in order to come home and assume her unwanted inheritance.

'And then creeps like this come in,' she complained to the policeman. 'Charge him.'

Hugh, unused to being a criminal, claimed he was just carrying the coffee maker to the cash. He insisted he had been about to pay for it. The policeman convinced the owner to accept this solution, stayed at the cash register while Hugh paid, then accompanied him outside. Hugh gave an embarrassed handshake and then, arms around the split tennis bag and the $450 coffee maker, walked home. Its weight was impressive, also the fact that he had his arms around something.

The next day Hugh sewed up the bag and went to collect some more entries. He settled down with them – and a cup of excellent cappuccino – in one of his red Salvation Army armchairs. 'The first lines are the giveaway,' Hugh always said. The first entry he picked up began: *My aunt had one leg longer than the other which is why she always made a strange noise walking in high heels.* Hugh dutifully read through to the end, although perhaps skipping the odd line or page.

The next entry started off with a warning: *This may not be a memoir, but I do remember that I fell in love with Joshua when the snowmobile we were riding on tipped over and he landed on me.*

The third commenced with a joke Hugh hadn't heard for a few years: *The flowers growing outside our house would wilt in the fall, but my father always had spring in his step.*

Hugh lost consciousness during a description of a family Christmas dinner, but rebounded sufficiently to stagger from the chair – where previous naps had given him a stiff neck – to the couch, where he was gone for good.

When he woke up, he could feel his blood running through his veins like barking dogs. 'My blood is running through my veins like barking dogs,' Hugh said aloud. He paid off the dogs with another cup of cappuccino. Then he went into the bathroom to prepare for the book launch he was to attend that evening. He had noticed that one of the side-effects of celibacy, since leaving Sarah, was that he always seemed to be either shaving or brushing his teeth.

He stood in front of the mirror, contemplating his shaving cream. Generously spread, it looked like a Santa Claus beard. Suddenly Hugh wanted matching hair. A few more squirts and his head was also covered in rippling white lather. With his glasses, creamy white hair and beard, Hugh looked better to himself than he had for a long time.

With the first swipes of the razor, he exposed his right cheek. He used the lather gained to give himself white eyebrows. It was easy to see that all this shaving cream provided a terrific improvement on his normal situation: thinning dark hair, sparse eyebrows, cleanshaven face.

Hugh contemplated the romantic life he might be having

with thick white hair, a white fluffy beard, matching eyebrows. The other day he had been down at the CBC, picking up memoirs and having coffee with two fellow judges, Marlene and Kelly. They had just finished sharing a book on menopause and were discussing how unhelpful men were during this crisis in women's self-esteem. 'What about men's self-esteem?' Hugh had asked. Predictably, they laughed.

Hugh stepped into the shower. His Santa Claus costume fell to his shoulders, slid down his legs then hovered briefly at the drain, shrinking before it disappeared.

In better days Hugh would have imagined it reconstituting itself on the various sewer rats, mutated eels and dwarf crocodiles that swarm beneath the city, feeding on garbage and harbour worms. But Hugh's mind had slipped elsewhere, to one of the losing memoirs he was unable to lose. Despite the rules of the contest it was fifty pages in length, which was over twice the maximum allowed. It wasn't even typed – instead it had been written by hand with a fountain pen in the sky-blue ink Hugh himself used to favour. The letters were large but poorly formed, often straying from their assigned lines and also occasionally blotched by what Hugh assumed were tears.

'The Death of My Father' described how the writer, a woman in her late fifties and supporting herself and her alcoholic husband by working as a nursing assistant, felt about her father's recent death. *My father died two weeks ago. I cried but I was not sad for him.* The memoir then went on to describe how the father had beaten the woman as a child, deserted the home, then returned decades later, dying, to ask for help. Because it did not conform to the rules, Marlene and Kelly had said it would be unfair to consider it along with the others. But instead of simply sending it back with the form rejection slip, they had recommended a personal note reminding the woman of the regulations.

Reading the memoir Hugh had recognized the refrain he'd

finally deciphered from Sarah: manhood, even if unable to inflict pleasure, still guarantees pain. In other words, as he'd once said back to her, Men are cruel beasts who, purposefully or not, harm and deform everyone with whom they come in contact. It's not their fault, she'd conceded, it was all a matter of history and genetically induced tyranny.

The party was to launch a book called *Speak Up!*, the memoirs of a wealthy theatre patron, Anthony Millen. Its opening line was, *I always had the loudest voice in the class.* Hugh received two invitations. The first was sent from the publisher's publicity department – his status as contest judge had brought him this small perk. The second was from Millen himself – with the word *Finally!* scrawled across it by hand. This because Hugh ('more than a judge, less than a jury,' he would say to Sarah) had helped to write the book, in fact had constructed it from taped interviews and newspaper clippings. The proceeds had supported Hugh during his time in Paris.

When he arrived at the party, Millen came up right away. 'What have you got to tell me?' he boomed into Hugh's ear. This had been his standing greeting for the taping sessions. Across the living room Hugh spotted a table set up as a bar, surrounded by some familiar faces. As he moved towards it, steel fingers wrapped around his arm.

It was the woman from the hardware store. 'Excuse me,' she started, 'I wanted to tell you that I'm sorry about the other day. I felt terrible about it afterwards.'

The light was so strong Hugh could see a fine line of blonde hairs along the woman's upper lip. Recently he had developed a habit – embarrassing even to himself – of intently staring at women in public, soaking up those details best noted in intimate situations. He knew he shouldn't do this but he couldn't help himself – it was his only remaining female contact. Finally he stammered out, 'Really – I just – .'

The woman's fingers tightened. 'I was going to write you and apologize,' Hugh lied. He patted her fingers, to remind them what they were doing.

'My name is Carolyn.'

'Hugh Thurman.'

'Yes, I know. I looked it up on your credit slip. *I* was going to write *you*.' She loosened her grip, her arm dropped back to her side. Dressed up, elegant, chestnut hair renewed, she looked *substantial* compared, for example, the only example he had, to Sarah. Hugh offered to get her a drink. At the bar he sank into other conversations. By the time he had a glass of wine in hand for Carolyn, he saw she was surrounded and drinking already.

As Hugh left the party Carolyn smiled at him across a conversation and Hugh felt an unfamiliar tug. The next morning, when he switched on his kitchen lamp it exploded. He took it down to the hardware store. An assistant asked him to leave it for a few hours. When he returned later that afternoon, Carolyn took him to the back office and rewired the lamp while he watched her steel-band fingers weave their way swiftly through the electrical intricacies. To see better what she was doing, Carolyn put on a pair of granny glasses. Bent over her lamp she looked like a mother, sewing. Hugh found himself inspecting her fingers for rings. On her right hand she was wearing a narrow gold band.

The golden light from her ring soaked her fingers, her hands, her arms and throat. Hugh's mind made a little loop. He pictured her at the *Speak Up!* party – yet could not remember anything out of the ordinary about her skin.

She turned to look up at him. Again, under the bright light the colour in her eyes broke apart. Again Hugh did a re-run of the party. There, he was certain, her eyes had been brown. He imagined himself writing a memoir about this woman, this

Carolyn. *It all began with her skin*, he would begin. But after that?

Carolyn seemed to be waiting for him to speak, but Hugh's mind could do nothing but fold deeper into itself. Now he remembered how he walked home after the party, telling imaginary stories to an imaginary psychiatrist. Wet snow was falling when he left the party, but by the time he arrived home the snow had turned to sleet and Hugh's coat was soaked through.

To warm up, he had made some coffee in his machine, then added rum for reasons of health. He repeated this formula until, in a state of jellied depression, he'd stumbled into bed and dreamed the party. In the dream everything was as it had been until he saw that Millen was wearing a fluorescent blue bikini swimsuit.

In the dream, Carolyn was not dressed for swimming. She had on a white satin slip. Her skin glowed through and around it, and she kept pressing herself against Hugh.

'I used to know her father,' Millen confided loudly. 'We went whoring on the Nile together.'

'Is this for the book?' Hugh asked.

Millen laughed.

Then Hugh had looked at himself. His feet were dead pale, except for his toes, even more deformed than usual, with red patches and bruised-looking nails.

'Have you been kicking something?' Carolyn asked.

'Himself,' Millen supplied.

Dinner started as a beer across the street, because by the time Carolyn had finished the shop was otherwise closed and Hugh found himself saying, as though nothing could be more natural, 'Could I offer to buy you a drink?' Even pronouncing these innocent words made Hugh break out into a sweat.

'I was supposed to go out with my sister tonight.' But before Hugh could know if he was relieved or disappointed, Carolyn had punched her sister's number into the telephone. An answering machine came on. 'This is a message for Sally,' Carolyn began, and went on to say she was cancelling because of a headache. Carolyn brushed against Hugh as she turned from the telephone. After the breakup, Sarah had performed a post mortem on the remains of his psyche, her tongue serving as scalpel. During this inquest Sarah's indictment featured the accusation that Hugh was incapable of pure friendship – meaning, Hugh knew, the avoidance of certain damp experiences best forgotten. 'I will be a truly pure friend to Carolyn,' Hugh resolved to himself. Although, so far, all he'd done was to try stealing a $450 coffee maker.

The first awkward beer was followed by a second. Carolyn's skin retained its golden tones. Hugh relaxed. Carolyn played with her hair. The way her fingers kept nervously gathering and releasing made her seem oddly vulnerable, like a certain kind of female character in an old-fashioned play. She ordered more beer and more french fries. She talked about long division, and then about the time her sister had to wear a cast for six months. She twirled the ring on her finger but she didn't say anything about it. Hugh was about to ask but, every time he had his mouth open to speak, Carolyn held up a french fry and fed it to him. Hugh let himself float along. On the third beer the gold began to take on a certain flush. Carolyn fed him more french fries, sliding them gently onto his tongue. Carolyn was still talking, now about a trip to New Orleans. Hugh found this infinitely relaxing. Being a friend wasn't so difficult. He drank more beer to wash away the new round of french fries. He realized he would like, in a purely friendly way, to be in a bedroom with Carolyn. He would be lying down, attached to an intravenous supply of beer. She would be talking and feeding him. He would close his eyes. Still talking she would enclose him. Life would be perfect. Morning would never come.

They stayed drinking until closing time, having switched from beer to scotch. By this time Carolyn was sometimes forgetting the french fries when she put her hand to Hugh's mouth, and Hugh would run his tongue along her offered fingers. They had a sweet, salty taste, and as he licked his lips Carolyn would smile at him complicitly. When the tavern lights blinked, Hugh stood up and said, 'I could make you coffee.'

Hugh led her up the fire escape. 'I like music,' Carolyn announced, and walked through the kitchen, past the coffee maker to the living room.

Hugh went to the bathroom. He realized that despite the beer and the scotch, he was not yet drunk. Relaxed, yes, but not drunk. But he could still taste the beer and it mixed unpleasantly with the left-over taste of the french fries. He splashed his face with water, then brushed his teeth. 'At least I'm not shaving,' Hugh said to himself, but no one was listening.

By the time Hugh got back to the living room, Carolyn had put on an Ella Fitzgerald tape. She was standing in the middle of the room, chewing gum and swaying slowly to the music. Her inviting smile. Her golden skin in the lamplight.

A line from the abused woman's memoir offered itself: *My father would always turn on the radio and then ask me to dance. It was as though he was asking me to forgive him. I could never refuse him.*

Hugh went to stand beside Carolyn. She held out her hand. He took it. She swayed closer to him. Hugh swayed with her. Carolyn moved in closer, fitted herself to him. Her lips on his neck. Her hand holding his back. As though they were dancing the last dance at some long-ago prom. Sarah had been so thin, so elusive. Carolyn seemed so substantial, so willing. Hugh let his own arms fold around Carolyn. For a moment she seemed to stiffen. He hesitated. Then she moved in again.

Her breasts were heavy on his chest, her hands sliding up and down his back. As she danced them past the lights, she turned them off.

When the room was dark she turned her face up to be kissed. As their lips met, Hugh wondered what had happened to her gum.

Her heavy breasts. The way she was starting to breathe. The way she was rotating slightly as they danced, rubbing him with unmistakable intent.

They bumped into the couch. Carolyn dragged him down. With no warning, Hugh burped. It brought the taste of beer and fries back into his mouth. He turned his head away from Carolyn. 'Here,' she whispered. She was pressing something into his hand. Hugh began unwrapping it, thinking it was the minty gum he had been tasting on her lips. Then he realized it was a condom. 'I'll do it,' she whispered. Before Hugh knew it, his pants were down and Carolyn's expert hands were guiding him to the desired destination.

Events overtook themselves, but Carolyn murmured sweetly, and as they stumbled from couch to bedroom, she held him tightly. They fell onto the bed. An unpleasant taste rose to his mouth, but as he was thinking of going to brush his teeth, Carolyn wrapped her arms around him and Hugh, surprised and comforted, fell asleep.

Morning found Hugh kneeling over Carolyn.

'Hurry up,' Carolyn said.

Her skin, golden in this morning light. She pressed herself against him, a tawny welcoming golden goddess. Hugh hovered over her, looking down at her body. He had never dared to hope he could be wanted by someone this beautiful, this voluptuous.

'Kiss me,' she commanded. A shaft of light split open the colours of her eyes and he felt his own psyche, suddenly healed, re-born, splitting open with them. He looked down into the darkness where their bodies joined. The round welcoming swell of her belly. His own belly, white and furry. Carolyn's eyes were closed. Hugh felt suddenly calm and entirely at ease with himself, perfectly poised in time and space. For the first time in months he had absolutely no desire to shave or brush his teeth. In his memoirs, it came to him, he could describe this moment as the one fate had chosen to declare him a god. Then the taste of french fries rose again. As he turned his head to burp, Carolyn pulled him close. Suddenly Hugh's body jackknifed. As he sank into her, Carolyn moaned and Hugh began to vomit uncontrollably.

'It was the french fries,' he kept saying, 'you're the one who fed them to me.' But even as he babbled on, she was wrapping herself in a sheet. When he tried to touch her, she shoved him away. He fell backwards, grabbed something to cover himself. By then she had gathered up her clothes and slammed into the bathroom. 'Have a sense of humour,' Hugh pleaded through the door.

The next day, Hugh had to make a trip downtown to get another batch of memoirs. Before leaving the apartment he gave himself a lecture about the moral cowardice of fools. Every time he closed his eyes he tasted her fingers in his mouth, felt her pushing against him as they danced, saw her smooth golden belly arching towards his. Walking down the street he rehearsed alternative beginnings to his apology. When he got to the store Carolyn was standing in the doorway, the morning light on her face. 'I'm sorry,' Hugh began. Carolyn smiled tightly, stared at him for a moment. Hugh sank into her eyes. Everything was still possible. 'Go away,' Carolyn said.

On his way home, Hugh crossed the street to avoid walking in front of the store. A few weeks later, he moved.

some rules about adultery

catherine hiller

He was short, chunky, balding, bespectacled – not at all the kind of man Daria flirted with at parties. Yet here she was again, off in an intimate corner with Henry at another of Bettina's soirées.

Henry Pomeranz, a divorced professor of anthropology, was one of Bettina's old boyfriends. Daria had known him a little for years and thought he was intelligent, cultured, goodhearted – and nerdy. So it always amazed her how a few words from him could make her shine and blush.

In their alcove, Henry said, 'I like you with your hair like that. It's nice to see the shape of your face.'

Daria had put her hair up with a barrette because of the heat of the party. Now she could feel that some of the hair in the back had come down. Thick strands lay on her neck, like limp lily leaves. She said, 'It's falling.'

'I'll put it back up for you."

She looked past him in their alcove and into the rest of the room. She couldn't see her husband, Lewis.

Daria and Lewis had been married twenty years. She was forty-three, with large brown eyes, a wide jaw, and a slender body; she had often been told she looked like a dancer. He was tall and lean, clean-shaven, so you could see all the beautiful bones in his face.

In the next room, people were dancing. Daria thought Lewis was probably there.

'I'm good with hair,' said Henry, coming closer.

Daria said nothing. Henry opened the barrette, and her hair tumbled down. He watched it fall, then ran his fingers from her scalp to the ends of her hair. Again and again, he moved his fingers through her hair, as if combing it out. She stayed very still, because his hands on her head and along her hair were like hot winds running down her body. Her head drooped, like an overblown rose, and he gathered her hair and gently tugged it upward to look at her. Then he let all her smooth hair fall to her shoulders again. 'Have to start over,' he murmured, and she felt every tendril glowing yes toward him.

'I must be very drunk,' she lied, closing her eyes and drifting into space under his hands.

'What's going on here?' asked Bettina.

Daria opened her eyes. The good thing was, Henry didn't stop fiddling with her hair so nothing seemed covert and she could keep on enjoying his touch. Now that her eyes were open, Daria found that she could think and she could talk. She said to Bettina, 'Henry's being good enough to help me with my hair.'

He clipped the barrette closed and said, 'That should do it.' In parting, he gave the back of her neck a short, transcendent caress.

'Wow,' said Bettina. 'How long has this been going on?'

Henry Pomeranz replied, 'It's just beginning, isn't it, Daria?'

'*What?*' Daria felt stupid, speechless, both ways dumb, pink with shame and joy. How could he know her excitement? She had been so quiet.

'I'm getting another glass of wine,' he said, grinning, moving past them. 'Can I get you anything?'

The women shook their heads. When he had gone, Bettina said to Daria, 'Are you interested?'

Daria said nothing.

'I know he thinks you're hot.' Bettina tossed her dark hair back and looked into Daria's eyes. Bettina's eyes glowed turquoise. She said, 'You might be great together.'

Since Bettina's marriage to Bernie the year before, she and Henry had become the best of friends. They walked and took bike-rides together. He babysat for her little son. He told her all about his love-life. If Henry had an extra ticket, he would take Bettina to a concert or the theater. He and Bernie went to basketball games together.

'Really,' said Bettina, managing to speak *sotto voce* over the noise of her party, 'you should think about it with Henry.'

Swaying slightly from the afterglow of Henry's hands, Daria wondered why Bettina was urging him on her. Perhaps she wanted to be in the middle, the confidante of both.

Daria found herself saying to Bettina, 'This is not a good time for me to have an affair. Lewis and I have been quarreling.' As a long-married woman with a sulky daughter of sixteen, Daria sometimes enjoyed shocking her newly-married friend. Now Daria pronounced, 'I would only start an affair if things were going well with Lewis.'

When it came time to leave, Daria looked for Henry so she could say goodbye and give this stubby man an excuse to lay hands on her again, but she couldn't find him anywhere.

Three weeks went by before Henry Pomeranz called. By then, Daria had almost forgotten about his hands on her hair, and she and Lewis had stopped fighting. When things were going well at work, Lewis became altogether better-natured. Once again, it was clear to Daria that she and Lewis had a strong and happy marriage, so she agreed to meet Henry at the Museum of Modern Art the following Tuesday.

Daria had some rules about adultery. She would never fool around with a friend or an associate of Lewis's. She never made a date unless Lewis was at work so she could say to herself that she wasn't depriving him of anything, really. And she always hid her trysts without ever having to lie. As a fundraiser for a large theater company, Daria spent hours away from the office seeing people. She could easily spend time with a lover – although she hadn't done so since breaking up with Pierre two years before.

Now she had Tuesday to think about. Henry had told her that he didn't teach on Tuesday. God, would she soon know his schedule, his telephone number, and his apartment as well as she knew her own?

Meeting him at the Museum was initially deflating. He was shorter and plainer than she had remembered. He did not greet her romantically: he shook her hand hello. He was wearing a rumpled oxford shirt and blue jeans neither sexily tight nor fashionably baggy. She thought, this is a man with zero pizzazz.

They wandered through the permanent collection, pointing out their favorite paintings. They turned a corner and she said, 'Where's the Manet that was here?'

'I think it's out on loan.'

Daria said, 'They shouldn't take away my friends without consulting me.' She wondered if this didn't sound too cute, but he seemed charmed, he was smiling at her.

'They're better than friends,' he said, 'because they don't change. We never want our friends to change, do we?'

This had not occurred to her, and seemed true, and she looked at him thoughtfully.

'How long were you married?' she asked suddenly.

'Eighteen years. And I've been divorced five. Are you happily married?'

'Mostly.'

'We had an open marriage,' he said.

'I don't,' said Daria.

'I can respect that. Are you ready for some lunch?'

In the museum dining room, Daria told Henry a bit about her happy marriage. 'I always find Lewis interesting,' she said. 'And we enjoy our lives together. We're lucky, I guess.'

She did not tell him that over the course of her happy marriage she had also had four lovers. In her sudden conviction that she could never sleep with Henry because he wasn't good-looking enough, Daria said, 'Lewis is smart, he's dynamic, he's hard-working, and he's funny.'

'That's all very nice,' said Henry Pomeranz, 'but does Lewis worship your body?'

He put his hand on her forearm. A hot wind hit her chest and left her breathless, smiling wordlessly.

'What's so funny?' he asked.

'Lewis and I have passed the worship stage.'

'That's a pity,' said Henry. He grazed his fingers from her elbow to her wrist and then ran them lightly up again. He stuck his thumb deep into the inner crook of her elbow. Her arm, she now realized, had become an erogenous zone, and he was giving it to her, filling her up. Her breath came fast.

Henry smiled and withdrew his hand. 'Think about it,' he said. 'I have to go.'

'Yes, I have to go too.' Daria stood up with difficulty. She was insanely turned on. It made no sense. What did he have, anyway? Magic fingers?

After they parted – she insisted on putting her mouth upon his – she turned around to look at him. A short chunky man in a rumpled shirt was walking away from her with a bounce in his step.

Another of Daria's adultery rules involved a waiting period, so the following Tuesday, they met at the Brooklyn Botanical Gardens. The cherry blossoms were out – if a little past peak – and Daria and Henry walked on a carpet of petals.

'I wish you were married,' said Daria.

Henry asked, 'Why is that?'

'It would make it more even between us. We'd want the same things. I wouldn't worry about . . .'

'What?'

'Oh, things.' It seemed immodest to say she wouldn't worry about him falling in love with her – and premature to say she didn't want him single, out there, meeting other women. Married lovers were best for many reasons. Pierre had been married, and so had the other three.

Four affairs over twenty years wasn't so terrible, was it? Though Lewis would certainly think so, unless he'd had affairs of his own. She never asked. Either way, she knew, she'd feel bad.

'I'm not married now,' said Henry Pomeranz, 'but I know how it is. I'd be careful. I'm a player.'

His eyes looked small and glittery behind his thick glasses. He moved closer to her under the cherry blossoms. But instead of kissing her, he reached for her head. He pressed his thumbs in the space between her eyebrows and circled there slowly. The tips of his fingers played in her hair. She felt his strong, gentle hands soothing her, smoothing her, stroking her brain.

Daria had never known a man, married or not, with hands as good as this. She swayed against him. He patted her behind. Soon she felt she had a second brain down there.

'Next Tuesday,' he said, 'we'll meet in my apartment.'

Both her brains agreed.

'So what's going on between you and Henry?' asked Bettina at lunch the next day. They were in a coffee shop eating turkey sandwiches. Bettina taught English at a college near Daria's office.

'What does Henry say?' asked Daria.

Bettina said, 'He says he's seeing you, nothing more.'

'There's not much more to say.' Only Henry's hands on her for a few seconds here and there. 'He wants to "worship my body,"' Daria couldn't help adding. 'Maybe some day I'll let him.'

Bettina shook her head and frowned at her forkful of coleslaw.

Daria asked, 'What is it?'

'I thought I'd enjoy this more than I do.'

Daria grinned. 'That's life,' she said. 'Ever surprising. You didn't, I gather, find anything unusual about Henry's hands?'

Bettina shook her head again. 'I'll look at them next time I see him.'

Daria tried to recall what Henry's hands looked like. She smiled as she realized she hadn't a clue.

'You're no fun when you're like this,' grumbled Bettina. 'All grinning and silent. And Henry's the same way. Instead of knowing everything about your affair, or whatever it is, I know nothing!'

'People aren't puppets,' said Daria. 'You can't always pull all the strings.'

It was too warm for a jacket, so Henry couldn't help her off with anything, so he had no excuse to touch her on greeting. 'Hello, hello,' he said, grinning. He showed her his place. It was a pleasant apartment midtown. They ended the tour in the living room. A little feast was spread upon the coffee table near the couch. Small bowls held taramasalata, babaganoush, olives, dried figs, fresh strawberries, white cheese. Pita bread and Russian rye lay on a cutting board. There were two wine glasses and an open bottle of Beaujolais.

'Are you thirsty?' asked Henry, and she nodded and drank. Then she found herself eating voraciously. Henry sipped at his wine and watched her.

'So good!' she said. 'Delicious.'

She dipped a piece of pita into the babaganoush and pronounced, 'This is my favorite kind of eating. Little rich hors d'oeuvres.'

She reached for a dried fig. Would she ever stop eating? He wasn't making it easy by not touching her. If he wasn't going to touch her what was she doing here at all? She took a second fig.

'Do you always eat like this?' he asked with a smile.

'It's all so good. And maybe I'm nervous.' She considered what next to put in her mouth. She placed a chunk of cheese on a piece of rye and brought it to her lips. She took a bite.

'Don't be nervous,' said Henry, touching her forehead.

At once, eating was impossible. The bread and cheese turned to clay in her mouth. She spat them discreetly onto a napkin and turned toward Henry.

He tortured her. He stroked her head for ten minutes before doing anything else, and then he spent even longer massaging the back of her neck.

Hot, damp, trembling, Daria finally croaked, 'Maybe we should go to your bedroom.'

He chuckled. 'If you like.'

She took off all her clothes and lay on his white sheets awaiting him. He took off his clothes too. He had such a thick mat of hair on his chest it was like fur. His chest itself was round and soft around the nipples, so from a certain angle it looked like he had furry breasts.

This was Daria's last coherent thought for some time.

Paunchy Henry Pomeranz brought her bliss upon bliss.

Daria had always enjoyed making love with her handsome husband, and her previous lovers, but Henry pleased her more than anybody ever had. She wanted whatever he did, even if she'd never thought of it before.

He pinched her lightly down low.

He placed her legs in a strange position so that he and she made an x and their heads were far apart.

He wet his index finger and placed it where they were conjoined.

She moaned, she screamed, she wept.

Sometimes she looked at him. Invariably, his eyes were closed and he was smiling, Buddha-like, utterly serene, as if he'd found a sacred place.

In the next few weeks Daria noticed that in New York City there were many men who looked something like Henry. Whenever she saw one of his tribe, chunky men of middle age with beards, she would examine him closely and wonder about him in bed. Twice, she'd been startled when a Henry look-alike had returned her hungry gaze. Being in love with Henry left her open to a whole new range of men.

'What's going on?' asked Bettina one day on the phone. 'I've never seen Henry so happy.'

Daria gave a giggle.

Bettina said, 'What is it? Just sex?'

'Uh-huh.'

There was a pause, then Bettina burst out, 'I don't get it. I don't remember anything special about him!'

'I find him just perfect.'

'He's not real big or anything.'

'That's true.'

'And he's not all that virile.'

Their first afternoon together, Henry and Daria had made love four times. But she didn't want to compare notes with Bettina, so Daria just said, 'I'd rather be in bed with Henry Pomeranz than doing anything else in the world.'

'I don't believe this,' said Bettina in exasperation.

Daria had written poetry in high school and stories in college, and now she wrote grants as part of her job. But she had never before felt moved to write a myth, not even mentally. Now, during the slow times of her day, on the street or before sleep or in the car with Lewis, she was constructing a story to account for Henry's hands. For he was good with his mouth and good with his cock and good with positions and ideas. But he was utterly fantastic with his hands. And as she wondered why, she felt in her bones what she had learned theoretically at college: that mystery begets myth and that the need to explain fires fiction.

One afternoon at the office, Daria wrote down the myth she had made. She gave it to him on his birthday. As he read, a smile came and went upon his face.

In the myth, Henry arrives at his office early one morning and discovers a beautiful woman going through his files. Introducing herself as 'V,' she says she wants to read his notes on an ancient sex manual he is decoding. In return, she offers him a hand-drawn map of a township in Northern Ontario. She says, 'Bathe in the waters of this pond and you will always be happy in love.' 'Nonsense,' he says and starts to call Campus Security. She disappears, leaving the map. Three years later, on a whim, leaving for a lecture in Toronto, he brings along the map. He rents a car and drives to the pond. By then it is all silted over: there is no water to be seen, and wild grasses have grown over the wet field that once was a pond. Feeling rather foolish, Henry presses his hands to the soggy earth. Brown water bubbles around his fingers.

'After that,' Henry read, 'he could sleep with whoever he touched, for he brought utter joy to women with his hands.'

'How flattering,' said Henry. 'I suppose "V" is for Venus.'

'I suppose,' said Daria. 'Who else gave you this gift?'

'You gave me this gift,' he said. 'Don't you know?' And he took her in his arms. At moments like this, Daria thought she would lose her mind loving him.

Ninety minutes later, Daria showered and left. She went back to the office and worked for a couple of hours and picked up food for the family on her way home. For once her daughter wasn't sulking, and they had civil and interesting dinner conversation.

Her affair with Henry continued for two years. Daria awoke every morning and told herself what day of the week it was and thought about how far or near it was from Tuesday. Wednesday was okay because she had just seen him, and Thursday wasn't bad either. But Friday was terrible because by then she yearned for him again, and it was still *four days till Tuesday*.

Once again, as with Pierre and the others, Daria saw how deprivation heightens joy. But she had never been as crazed as this. By the time Tuesday came and she stepped off the elevator and walked down the hall to his apartment, just pushing his doorbell made her breathe fast. He would take her straight to the bedroom and she would whimper under his touch. He would find out soon how excited she was. 'Poor baby,' he would say pityingly.

Once when he just flicked her and she came, he looked down on her and laughed and laughed. And for the first time in her life she came twice in a row.

'God, are you hot,' he said, stroking her behind.

'Just with you.'

He ran his hand between her buttocks. He did a lot of that, and more, when they were making love. When she felt his finger poking into her like a fat thermometer, sometimes she'd push his hand away. It was the only thing he did she didn't love, and still she didn't really mind and would never have stopped him if she wasn't sometimes sore there later on.

Daria's favorite time with Henry wasn't really sexual. They were lying on the couch, fully dressed, both facing the ceiling. His head lay under her chin, and his back was on her belly. She put his hands on his forehead, holding him to her, adjusting her breathing to his. 'I'm so happy,' she said.

'So am I.'

Because she was married, they couldn't speak of love.

Perhaps he saw they'd reached a sort of limit and he wanted more. Perhaps he was frightened at how dependent on her he'd grown. Perhaps he had met a wonderful new woman. Each of these hypotheses seemed plausible to Daria. It was the third year of their affair, and Henry, while still avid for her body, seemed increasingly remote.

One Tuesday when she arrived, Henry gave Daria a pat intended to appease, not arouse. He said, 'We have to talk.' He steered her to the living room, where the food was laid out as usual.

'What is it, Henry?' Daria asked. They didn't usually get to the food for some time.

'I don't tell you much about my other life,' he said. 'My life between Tuesdays.'

'That's true,' she said. 'And Bettina certainly keeps mum.'

'At my request,' said Henry.

Daria sat on the couch. 'Are you serious about someone? Is that it?'

Henry paused just a moment before nodding.

Daria managed to say, 'Well, that's okay. I mean, I've got Lewis.'

'She wants to get married,' said Henry.

'Gee. What do you want?'

'I want to give it a chance. But every Tuesday afternoon there's you. And it's always so incredibly intense.'

Daria nodded.

Henry continued. 'Somehow, it isn't fair to Cindy.'

'Cindy!' Tears sprang to Daria's eyes as she said, 'What a wimpy name.'

'She's not a wimp at all.'

'I don't want to know about her.'

'I'm sorry,' said Henry. 'I think we should cool it for a while.'

'You mean, no more Tuesdays?'

He nodded.

'And today?'

'We'll eat, talk, drink some wine. Daria, every week when you rang the bell, I'd thank God for the hours ahead. I've loved every minute of our affair. But it couldn't last forever.'

'Not forever,' she said, trying to smile, 'but I thought perhaps another dozen years.'

He touched her neck, with the usual result. She said, 'How can I stop wanting you?'

'You just will.'

Daria shook her head. 'I'll be longing for you for the rest of my life.' She laughed to make it a joke.

He put both hands on her upper arms. 'Daria – what can I do?'

'Break up with Cindy,' she said promptly.

'Seriously,' said Henry, stroking her arms so they seemed to flicker with warmth from within.

The trouble is, Daria thought, there's this pairing for me –Henry and ecstasy. I have to break that link.

'Henry,' she said slowly, 'I think you should, I mean we should – somehow you and I have to have . . . bad sex.'

'What?' His fingers stopped moving on her arms.

Daria said, 'Then I won't feel so sad that you're breaking up with me.'

'One bad time will do it?'

'I think maybe three. Can you give me today and two more times?'

He hesitated.

She said, 'Never mind about you and Cindy! You also owe something to me.'

'Of course I do. But, Daria. How on earth are the two of us going to manage bad sex?'

She thought a bit and told him some things.

Henry said, 'It doesn't sound like fun.'

She said, 'That's the point. Come on, Henry, please.'

So they went into the bedroom to have some bad sex.

'No, no!' she said soon when they were on the bed naked. 'You're not supposed to do the things I like!'

'But I like them too.'

'Please. Not now. Remember what we're doing.'

Henry cupped her breasts and asked, 'Can't I even do this?'

She knew he could quietly hold them for minutes on end, varying the pressure infinitesimally while she sighed and moaned. 'Have mercy,' said Daria. 'No foreplay. Come in.'

'If you insist,' he said, entering her. He began one of his slow, delicious strokes.

'Not like that!' Daria said. 'Fast and hard, like a jackhammer.'

His rhythm grew fast, he shut his eyes tight. A grimace contorted his face.

She squeezed him encouragingly. Although she didn't like this staccato rhythm she'd commanded, if he didn't come soon, she just might. She touched him again, and he shuddered mightily. Then he was still. His weight was heavy upon her. He seemed to have fallen asleep. She tried to ease out from under him, but he wouldn't let her leave.

'My darling,' he murmured, stroking her head. She saw it hadn't been all that bad for him.

'None of that, Henry,' said Daria, slipping away from his embrace. She knew how afterplay became foreplay with him. 'I have to go.'

'So soon?'

'It's best.' She had to leave dissatisfied. 'See you next Tuesday for more.'

'Are you sure about all this?' He put on his glasses and sat up in bed. His furry tits sagged.

'Oh, I am,' said Daria. 'It's working already.'

'Hello,' Henry said enthusiastically the next week. He fingered her blouse. 'Nice silk.'

He guided her toward the bedroom. 'Remember, bad sex,' she reminded him, for he was touching her neck.

'Of course.'

'Could you be utterly passive today? Just lie there like some effete king?'

'I guess so. You mean, I'm not supposed to do anything?'

'Nothing at all.'

'If you insist.'

He lay flat on his back on the bed. She had to push his hands off her breasts when he forgot his instructions, and when she went lower, she twice removed his hands from her head. Then she moved up on his body and sat down on him hard, jamming it in. She rode vigorously up and down. She kept her eyes open and watched. She saw how he gasped at the end: 'Daria, Daria, Daria!'

She was unmoved by any of it.

Daria thought about canceling her third session. After all, she was probably already free from Henry's spell. She needed only one more treatment for her cure – and it held no appeal for her at all.

As Daria sat by the phone, she vowed she would never let anything like this happen again. Never again would she sleep with an unmarried man! That would be another adultery rule. Besides, there was health to consider. Henry had tested HIV negative, he had told her, but did he *keep* getting tested? And what about Cindy?

When Daria called to break her last date with Henry, she

got his answering machine. At the sound of his voice, she felt swollen below, so she guessed she wasn't quite over him yet. She left no message and appeared at his door the next Tuesday as usual.

Past Henry's shoulder, she saw the small plates and bowls in the living room. She found she was very hungry, especially for some wrinkled black olives (although she knew they'd make her breath bitter). She gazed longingly at them.

But Henry was taking her into the bedroom for her final treatment. 'One second,' she called, breaking free from him. She scurried into the living room and prepared a plate for herself – olives, fresh mozzarella, and peppers. She sat down on the couch with it and he sat next to her. He broke some bread off a long loaf for himself and ate it dry, watching her, bemused.

'Any special instructions?' he asked. 'For the bedroom?'

She nodded grimly.

'Well?' he asked.

'Try to guess.'

He made a gesture and she nodded. She asked, 'How did you know?'

'It's just about the only thing we haven't done – you never seemed to want to. Are you ever going to finish eating?'

'I'd like another glass of wine, thank you.'

Henry groaned. Daria smiled. It was fun to call the shots, and she needed the wine, and she stayed in the living room as long as she could.

Finally they went into the bedroom. Soon, she wished she was drunker. She had never loved Henry, she thought while he made love to her as if she was a boy. It was painful, and ugly, and she wouldn't miss him one bit.

He gripped her buttocks savagely and screamed.

Moments later, he eased out of her, and soon after that, he was asleep, smiling slightly, like a Buddha. She held him in her arms one final time. Then she looked at her watch and pulled away.

He opened his eyes and smiled. 'What's your hurry?'

'I have to be back at two for a meeting.'

He stroked her arm, and all along her nerves and muscles, her cells felt magnetized.

'Don't, Henry,' she said. 'It would spoil everything.' She stood up near the bed.

'We have to talk,' he said. 'I've been thinking. Maybe we can still manage Tuesdays. At least until Cindy moves in.'

'I don't think so, Henry.' She thought, I couldn't do this twice.

She closed the bathroom door and had a long shower and washed every bit of it out of her.

When they parted, she said, 'See you later,' the ultimate inaccurate banality.

Bettina and Daria were having lunch at the coffee shop three weeks later. Bettina said, '*You're* doing fine. Since you and Henry broke up.'

'I suppose. I devised this weird cool-down program for us. I think it really worked.'

Bettina hesitated. Finally, she said, 'For you, maybe – not for him.'

'Oh?'

'He won't explain it, but he seems to be obsessed with you. He's still seeing Cindy – but he talks about you all the time.'

Daria felt her eyes sting with tears – whether for Henry or herself she didn't know. She kept her eyes down, so Bettina wouldn't see.

Bettina said, 'He can't believe you broke up with him when you did.'

Daria asked, 'How do you mean?'

'He said, "Not after all that incredible sex!"'
Through her tears, Daria burst out laughing.

It was three years before Daria took another lover. He was good-looking and married, and the sex wasn't bad.

dionysus day

alison fell

So what is she? This Aileen. The hair mice-tails, the face
   pastry-pale, but in the eyes, thank God, the wild fire of
   intelligence.
Don't carve on the desk Aileen he says, though he'd as
   soon not.
Rather wait and catch her out, fetch her to the Headmaster.
What she needs.
Pinky poking itself into the keyhole in his desk, I ask you.
What she does. Out at the front with her essay when he's
   talking to her. Pinking and poking at the wee hole. So
   wee.
Yes sir she says.
Kiss his ruler if she doesn't watch out, he'll show her.

Splinters. What light does when dust floats in it or despair.
He knew a teacher once who terrified. Touched his lips to
   his six-foot ruler, solid teak.
Bitter with the love of it. So that none watching and none
   listening could forget ever after that slight sighing smack,
   that glittering kiss.
A man who wanted to enter rooms like the sun and there's
   the shame of it.

Not that our Aileen knows anything of waste or shame.

See her out at the far frosty edge of the playground, one
    foot on the perimeter fence. Far it is she'll go, you can
    tell by the distance in the eyes.
Praise or blame it's all the same to Aileen. Clever Aileen
    whose one look can cut you to the heart.

Winter melts off the slopes of the mountains and the firs at
    the lochside are horizontal cliffs of light.
Up at the blackboard the chalk dust swirls like a mist.
Supercilious, he says. Spell that one madam. *Exhibit* your
    powers to us. One dress after another slipping over her
    head and clinging to his face like cobwebs. Shadows of
    rubbed-out words wavering under the new inscription.
    Shadows on her skin.
He touches the ruler to the board where the sun comes and
    goes.
Sir? says she, squinting.

Come summer he takes them up Ben Vorlich for the bike
    trials.
The mud torn by tyre-tracks, splattered hay-bales hanging
    off the edge of the path.
Midges too, but does our Aileen get a move on?
Oh no not she, not our wee Queen of the May.
Dawdle she does, her with the long legs and young, her
    with the hair in her eyes.
I'm awful tired sir.
The sun sweating down through the branches and he with
    the heat in his head and she on the path above him and
    the rest of them even higher.

Thinks she's a bird does she? Flies into the yellow bus after
    school with a kick of her heels but she'll not fly for him.
A dancer for a mother too.

These women with their skirts like white bells, the way they
    sway up and down on their tippy toes with their little
    black-laced feet and their fingers pointed out like
    princesses and their long scarves all the colours.
Practising.
A circle of white and the rustle of the long legs.

He knew a teacher once with a hook for a hand, she doesn't
    know when she's lucky.
She hanging wide-armed from an alder bush like a
    stretched cobweb.
I can't sir.
His shame that the rowan branch breaks so softly from the
    tree, rowan fit for a May Queen. Whippy and mean it is
    but spare the rod and so on.
All the cheating white meadowsweet banked up by the path
    to smother him.

And what does she do but start to cry. This Aileen with the
    bottom lip like a dinner plate. Surly face making her
    plain.
Now one look at Aileen and you'll agree she could fly away
    if she wanted, could've been at the top with the rest and
    long since.
But does she?
Hot the fly-laden moments in the heather as he laughs at
    her.
On and up Aileen.
Laughs loud for joy at the high fine day it is and suddenly
    the birds singing, full May by the blether of the waterfall
    and he with his darling, her skin white as the pith of the
    reed, her skin milk-white under the dusty flower of the
    rowan.

Sprawling, her eyes plead. Shadows in the love-grove.
He'll give her green under the eyelids and a goatskin to lie
   on.
Oh his flower trampled in the dirt.
On and up, my darling.
But will she?
Oh his love he'll give her a toffee apple on this toffee apple
   day which began so red and crisp to the teeth and now
   the luscious noon of it waiting to be sucked up.

The words pouring from his mouth like leaves.
You know what it means Aileen. You know what it means
   when a woman dreams of painting a room red.

Say nothing. A finger to his lips.
White bone.

We all pay blood-money for what we've become.
Blood for believing we could escape. Blood to the sad hills
   and the fences. Blood to the women of youth and the
   smell of soup and the toil of the fireside.

Say nothing. His hands locked tight at his neck.
Oh the peck of her sharp teeth, his love, his silence.
Oh the kiss glittering.

At full noon, frantic, he creeps under the leaves.
The sun holds tight to his skull and the bright birds
   squabble above him.
And here they come now with their white scarves and their
   white teeth and their hair black and russet and yellow,
   here they come like a string of blossoms.

calendars
of the heart

scott bradfield

'Actually, all I'm looking for is great sex and someone who likes to stay up watching late-night movies on Cable TV,' Roland Simpson said, leaning earnestly across Dr. Sheidley's highly-organized mahogany desk. Dr. Sheidley was applying soft, sooty marks to a reddish computer card with a yellow Ticonderoga Number 2 pencil. 'I realize that doesn't sound like a lot to ask for from a relationship, but to me, well, I guess it really *is* a lot to ask. Sure, on rare occasions I've known women who were great in bed, but then it invariably turned out they weren't *sincerely* interested in old movies. On the other hand, the women I meet who like old movies are invariably lousy in bed. Go figure.'

Dr. Sheidley was a thirtyish, brunette, theoretically quite attractive woman with just about the sourest disposition Roland had ever encountered in a woman he wasn't currently dating.

'Preferred skin coloration?' Dr. Sheidley asked, her pencil poised like a scalpel.

'Doesn't matter,' Roland said.

'Height, weight, hobbies, special interests?'

'Doesn't matter,' Roland said.

'What about political or religious affiliations? University education or prior marriages? Smoker or non-smoker?'

'Doesn't matter,' Roland said. 'Doesn't matter, doesn't

matter, doesn't matter, doesn't matter. Like I was saying
–great in the sack, and likes to stay up late watching Cable TV.
I get HBO and Cinemax, but I'm willing to change. I'm willing
to grow *into* a relationship, if you know what I mean.'

Dr. Sheidley held the upraised pencil in her hand. She had a
very hard little face, Roland thought. But that didn't mean it
wasn't a rather hard little pretty face as well.

With a peremptory snap, Dr. Sheidley replaced her pencil in
the segmented plastic tray. She removed her Banlon tinted
eye-glasses and, for the first time that afternoon, Roland
found himself gazing directly into Dr. Sheidley's resoundingly
blue eyes.

'Are you putting me on, Mr. Simpson?' Dr. Sheidley asked
with a little rasp in her voice. 'Because if you are, I don't have
any time for it today.'

Dr. Sheidley looked especially pretty when she was angry,
Roland thought.

'No, Dr. Sheidley,' Roland said, smiling as politely as he
could. 'I'm not trying to put you on at all.'

'It took me years to realize it, Roland, but do you want to
know what my problem is? Well, if you're prepared for a little
brute honesty over the next few minutes or so, I'm going to tell
you.'

Wendy Steiner was an attractive, very available young
woman who was listed in Dr. Sheidley's Personal Contact
Portfolio as Account Number S (for Steiner) 0108. Earlier
that evening, she and Roland had met for the first time at
Stan's Seafood Restaurant in Sepulveda.

Wendy said, 'Don't tell anybody where you heard this,
Roland, but I happen to be one of those women who love too
much. I smother men with kisses and affection from the first
moment I see them until the last moment they fall asleep at
night. I cook them exorbitant, fatty meals and make love to

them at every conceivable opportunity in a storm of passionate frenzy which one former lover of mine used to characterize
as "excessive." Loving a man too much is just about the worst
thing you can do to him, since the male-ego is deeply terrified
of succumbing to oceanic female heterogeneity. Especially
these days.'

'Actually,' Roland said, reaching for his napkin, 'I'll bet
there are probably a lot of men out there who wouldn't mind
being loved too much. Me, for instance. Being loved too much
would probably suit me just fine.'

'No, Roland,' Wendy said, smiling patiently as if she were
confronted by a severely autistic child. 'You're just being nice
to me so you can get me into bed. Admirable strategy, Roland,
but that doesn't mean it's going to work. I've been out with
your type more than a thousand times before.'

'More than a *thousand*?'

'At the very least. Let's not fool ourselves, Roland. We're
both mature, fairly-enlightened single adults. We've both
been through the seventies and eighties, and now we're
prepared to explore single life in the strangest, most spiritually
fulfilling decade of them all. I'm talking about the Nineteen
Nineties, Roland. I'm talking about a decade in which mere
physical gratification isn't enough anymore.'

Roland glanced uneasily around the candle-lit restaurant
for the waiter, who had yet to return with Roland's third
White Russian. Politely Roland said, 'Actually, you know, I
never really dated that much in the seventies *or* the eighties. So
maybe I've got my share of physical gratification still coming
to me. Do you think life works that way?'

Wendy, however, wasn't listening.

'You want to know the *real* problem between men and
women, Roland?' Wendy had hardly touched her dinner
salad. She was hastily smoking one filter-tip cigarette after
another. 'Men are other-directed, and women are self-

directed. Men are other-directed because they have a penis, which is like this big arrow pointing *away* from the body. It's always pointing at other women, other places, other lives, *othernesses*. Territories of the unknown, the exotic, the unpollinated, and often the downright weird. This sort of penis orientation makes men incapable of being loved for very long without feeling deeply bored and claustrophobic. This is why men are always screwing every feminine-looking object that comes along, or disappearing for weeks on end drinking with their buddies and going to RV shows. Women, on the other hand, are much more self-oriented than that. Women are concerned with the inner essences and universal stabilities of things. They cherish permanent truths like love, family, home and hearth. Men are other-oriented because they have a penis, and women are self-oriented because they have a vagina, and I'm afraid there's absolutely *nothing* any of us can do about *any* of it. And Roland? If you don't mind my asking. Are you finished with your veal?'

Roland was still looking around the restaurant trying to locate his White Russian. He looked at Wendy. Then he looked at his veal. He was about half finished with his veal.

'Sure,' he said. 'I guess so.'

'Oh good,' Wendy said, with a long sigh of relief. 'Then maybe you could be a doll and drive me home. I've just come down with the most excruciating headache you could possibly imagine. However much I would *love* to watch Cable TV at your place.'

It was a deceptively sunny afternoon in early Spring when Roland returned home from his Color-Breathing Seminar to discover his estranged half-brother Albert urinating in the kitchen sink.

'You're not going to believe this, but it completely slipped my mind,' Albert confessed, fitting himself back into his Levis with an exaggerated little shrug of his shoulders. 'I been living, see, in this real Santa Ana rat-hole, where there's only this one toilet for the whole building? I guess it's gotten me into some real anti-social behavior strategies and all.'

Albert turned on the water and swung the faucet from side to side. Then he shut off the water and wiped his hands on the floral-patterned dish towel. 'It wasn't until I heard you come in the door that I realized. I mean, like I'm pissing in your kitchen sink and all. So how the hell are you, Roland? You're *looking* good, anyway. You're sure looking a damn sight better than you did the *last* time I saw you.'

The last time Albert saw Roland, Roland had been hurling Albert's Samsonite luggage down the front steps of his apartment complex.

Even though Albert was not noticeably any better-looking than Roland, he still managed to sleep with virtually all of Roland's girlfriends whenever he came to visit. Now, with Roland's female contacts at the Dating Institute proliferating daily, Albert set to work with the relentlessly disciplined abandon of an over-wound watch. He slept with Sarah F[eldman] 0108, Judy B[loomfield] 9007, Regina H[eadley] 0338, and even the lewdly disaffectionate Agnes P[ortobello] 8989. He slept with waitresses Roland customarily over-tipped, secretaries from Roland's office, and random women who shared anonymous time with Roland on neighborhood buses or in public laundromats. And of course the one woman Albert slept with the most often and with the most widely advertised success was Wendy Steiner, the one woman Roland loved more than any other woman in the entire world.

'Despite the fact your friend Wendy has a lot of crazy ideas about penises and vaginas and their effects on social behavior, she's quite a remarkable hellcat in bed, especially if you treat her really *lousy*,' Albert told Roland one night over a few friendly drinks. Having exhausted Roland's supplies of Glenlivet and Jack Daniels, Albert had ventured into the brighter domain of over-priced brandies and liqueurs. 'Being nice just doesn't work anymore. Okay, maybe it worked once upon a time for our stupid fathers and grandfathers, but that doesn't mean it's going to work for us. Women aren't materialistic like men are, Roland. Women know nice guys are a dime a dozen. They're not interested in boring old-fashioned things like security, fidelity, or even great hugs that past generations of women, blinded by the misogynist limitations of their socio-economic horizons, were uneducated enough to settle for quite happily. No, Roland, women today are looking for spiritual adventure, intellectual fulfillment, and really nice jewelry. I'm telling you, bro – treat Wendy lousy and she'll love you forever. Treat her like an object, and she'll hand you her heart on a silver platter.'

'But I *love* Wendy,' Roland said. A faint dizzy flush escalated into his face. 'I want to treat Wendy really *nice*.'

'Suit yourself, bro. But I'm on my way over to Wendy's right now for a steak dinner she's cooking – and that's not *all* she's cooking for me, bro. That's not all she's cooking for me by a long shot.'

Whenever Roland arrived home from work he could hear Albert screwing one of his former girlfriends with unabashed frenzy in the bedroom, transforming the headboard into a castanet and the wobbly end-tables into dominos. The living room floor was littered with cracker crumbs, wadded Kleenex and foil condom wrappers. The television and stereo were playing full blast, while 100 watt bulbs blazed indiscriminately in the halls and kitchen. Delivery-boys arrived every half hour or so with pizzas and buckets of chicken and demanded Roland pay for them. Albert, meanwhile, drank every ounce of liquor he could lay his hands on.

'I'm going to leave you with a little secret, Roland,' Albert said on the afternoon he lit out for parts unknown. Roland was at that moment once again hurling Albert's already well-dinged luggage down the front stairs of his apartment complex and watching the various pieces crash and leap on the white pavements, spilling everywhere the various clothes and possessions Albert had pilfered from Roland's bedroom bureaus and kitchen cupboards.

'Women aren't action, Roland,' Albert told him, 'they're *re*action, and that's the scary part. You see, men do stupid things because they don't know any better, but women are always trying *not* to do all the stupid things men *want* them to do. This makes women pretty goddamn confusing almost all the time. While men are busy trying to build bridges, eat fatty foods and design better mousetraps, women are trying not to be known, and not doing what they know men want them to do. Men spend their days banging at things, getting drunk, cursing, and digging bomb shelters in their back yards. Mean-while, women go journeying off into purely abstract territories, sitting on the sofa and looking a million miles away. By this point, problems between the sexes have gotten to be such a holy mess that the mere fact men have penises and women have vaginas doesn't really make things anymore confusing than they already are. By the way, Roland – did you really have to do that to my luggage?' Albert was smoking a fat Cuban cigar and buttoning the fly of his Levis. 'I may actually take the hint some day and stop visiting you altogether.'

'Is that my tennis racket?' Roland asked. The Samsonite overnight bag had exploded under the wheels of a swerving Toyota, and fragments of the shattered Wilson graphite racket landed in the driveway among a wide selection of Roland's newest silk ties and cotton-blend sports slacks.

'I'll be damned,' Albert said. 'I wonder how *that* got in there?'

*

Every time Roland attended one of Dr. Sheidley's Love-Attack Workshops, he invariably returned home suffering terrible headaches, or pinched nerves in his neck. He considered calling Wendy Steiner or one of his many female dating acquaintances from the Institute, but ever since Albert had disappeared into the mid-West selling silk flowers door to door, all of Roland's female acquaintances had sunk themselves into black clinical depressions, misuse of alcohol and barbiturates, and poor grooming habits.

'Women are the void,' Albert told Roland during one of his frequent trans-continentally collect phone calls. 'Women are the black dimensionless hiss of the holy eternal nothingness of the matterless unalphabeted void. Sound like bad Ginsberg, Roland? Well, it's not. It's hard merciless sexual reality, pal, and don't you forget it. You don't go trying to fill a dimensionless void, do you? You don't go tossing in roses, say, or bottles of aperitifs? There's no sense trying to fill a void because void is vacuum, absence, determinate indeterminacy, a whole lot of colorless nothing, pure indissoluble negation, anti-stuff, conceptual terrorism, Morpheus, Toronto, summertime in Detroit. You want to buy chocolates and roses for *that*, Roland? You want to hold *that* in your arms and whisper sweet nothings in *its* ear? Wise up, kid. If you want to make women happy, then first you got to know what they want. And you don't even know that much, do you, Roland? Try telling me, then. Try telling me just *one* thing women want.'

Roland's sweaty palm slipped against the plastic telephone receiver. He felt hot and panicky, and thought about pouring himself a nice large scotch. 'I don't know,' he said weakly. 'Love, happiness, a job they really like? What about money? What about a nice new car?'

'*Ha!*' Albert cried, as if he'd just discovered dynamite. 'You hopeless boob, Roland. *That's* what men *want* women to want

– that's not what women *really* want. Women want what men don't *want* them to want. Women want what men don't *want* them to have. It's simple logic, kid; we're talking your basic sexual dynamics here. Want, not-want. Take, not-be-taken. Desire, let's-not-*be*-desired. Flip and flop, flop and flip. I mean, you get a bunch of women together, Roland, and what do they talk about? What do women talk about when men aren't around?'

Roland started to hyperventilate. 'The weather?' he asked.

'No, Roland. And *try* paying attention to me for just one second, will you? When women get together, they talk about what they *don't* want. Who they don't want, and how badly they don't want to be wanted *by* them. Meanwhile, kid, what *do* they want? It's not such a trick question once you get the hang of it. What *do* women want, Roland? Flip and flop. Flop and flip.'

'What they . . . *want*?' Roland asked. The kitchen around him had gone stroboscopic and smoky, like a very bad disco. 'I mean, is what they . . . *want* what they want?'

'No no *no* no no no no, Roland, you breathless *turd*! You're not even listening to me! What women want – and you should probably write this down – is what they don't *not* want. They don't not want to be wanted by men who don't want them, for example.'

'I think I'm coming down with a migraine,' Roland said.

'That just means your brain's starting to work, kid. That just means you're starting to catch on.'

Roland felt hazy and vast, as if he were venturing into wide liminal spaces. 'So you're trying to say that . . . women want to not want what they don't not want?' Are these my words? Roland asked himself distantly. Are these my lips?

'*Exactly*, Roland!'

'What did I say?' Roland cried. 'What in God's name did I *say*?'

'And what *can't* they want, Roland?' Albert continued, as if he were urging a puppy through its first public handshake. 'You can do it, bro. What *can't* women ever *allow* themselves to want?'

'And . . . they *can't* want what they're not supposed to *not* want, but only if they're *not* supposed to want it?'

'*Now* you've got it, kid! Negation – pure indissoluble negation. And what do you do with pure negation, Roland – especially when you're staring into the vast white Godless heart of it? You ne*gate* it! Because that's the only choice you've got left anymore! You negate the negator!'

'Negate the negator?'

'That's it, Roland. Now you're cooking. Negate the negator. Will you do that for me, Roland? Negate the negator. Negate the negator, Roland. Ne*gate* the negator.'

'I will,' Roland said, feeling adrenalin lift into his chest and face. 'I will! I promise! I really will!'

'*Listen* to me, kiddo. Ne*gate* the negator! Make me proud of you! Ne*gate* the negator before *she* negates *you*!'

'I *won't*, then!' Roland cried, hurtling through different notions of distance now. 'I *won't*! I really, really *won't*!'

Roland canceled his subscription to all Dating Unlimited Self-Growth Support Services and disconnected his phone. He quit his job, sold his car and changed his name to Kevin Summerhall. He pulled the curtains, closed the blinds and nailed shut the front windows. Then he installed new burglar alarms throughout the house and garage and strung barbed wire around the backyard fences. He expanded his cable contract to include Bravo, The Movie Channel and the Home Shopping Network. Eventually, as the result of perseverance and hard work, a cloud of dull inactivity settled over Roland's life, as warm and protective as a shroud.

'I appreciate your concern, Dr. Sheidley,' Roland shouted

through the front door one morning. Dr. Sheidley had arrived on his porch carrying a briefcase filled with glossy brochures she hoped might tempt Roland back to his high-standing at the Dating Institute. 'But I think I've done enough dating to last a lifetime.'

Dr. Sheidley's voice held an unfamiliar little tremor, like a crack in an iron bell. Roland glimpsed her through the spy-glass. She was wearing a white silk blouse and sunglasses. 'Are you *sure*, Roland? It seems a terrible waste – you've been making such excellent progress and all.'

'And it probably *is* a terrible waste, Dr. Sheidley.' Roland was still pushing a few stray items of furniture against the heavily barricaded door. An end table. A stuffed chair. A box of books he was donating to Goodwill. 'But it's mainly a terrible waste of *your* professional training. I don't *deserve* your help, Dr. Sheidley. I'm a hopeless case and you shouldn't waste anymore of your valuable compassion on me.'

At night Roland could hear them, a slow gathering hush like whispering or respiration. Cars passed slowly in the street, flicking their high-beams on and off. Vague mournful faces appeared in the passenger windows, staring at Roland's front yard and porch. High-heels clacking on concrete, the raspy flare of sulphur matches, a scent of musk in the air. Sometimes he would turn the volume down on his television and just listen. The cold moon. Cold and hard.

'Look, Roland, we *miss* you, you big lug,' Wendy Steiner called from the front yard one night. 'Don't ask why. It's just chemistry, I guess. We miss seeing your stupid face at the Dating Lunches and Singles Dances. We miss that stupid little way you looked so hurt when we told you we didn't love you, and that we weren't *going* to love you, and when was your brother Albert coming back, anyway? It's crazy – sure. But so is romance, Roland. So is happiness. So why don't you come out for a little while and we'll go get a drink or something? No commitment, Roland – no kidding. We'll have a little drink together, and if you want to go home right afterward, that's fine with us.'

Wendy was standing in a pool of lamp light on the empty street, like an actress in a soliloquy. Roland peered into the hedges and alleyways where lumpish shadows gathered.

'Look, Roland,' Wendy said, tapping her foot impatiently on the sun-baked amber grass, 'I know I said a lot of rotten things about people with penises. And I'm sorry if my world-view tends to look at men as worthless scum. But that doesn't mean that in my own weird way I don't still *care* about you. Roland? Are you listening to me? Or are you going to hide in your house all night and sulk?'

Then one hot summer night way past midnight, Roland started awake in his bed. He heard it as distinctly as a footstep. A sudden lapse of energy, a break in the circuit.

Something had happened. Something had happened outside in the night.

Roland pulled on his robe and went to look out the kitchen window. Illuminated by high klieg lights Roland had mounted onto the encompassing fences, a dark shape lifted itself up and over from a neighboring yard and dropped onto the dead grass. Roland heard a cessation of crickets, twigs cracking. The hunched shape darted across Roland's back lawn with a piece of sharply glinting steel in its hand. Then the shape was leaning against Roland's picture window and fiddling at the lock with a long steel needle. Quick as a flash, Roland ran up beside the curtain. He stood poised with a large wooden axe-handle raised over his head. The axe-handle was reinforced with thick blue friction-tape. Roland had purchased both the axe-handle and the friction-tape only two days previously at House of Lumber in Tarzana.

After a moment, the lock on the picture window clicked resoundingly. The door screaked open on rusty aluminum casters, and the dark figure entered Roland's living room just as Roland cocked his shoulders against the weighty axe-handle.

'Yo, bro,' the dark figure said.

And not a moment too soon, Roland recognized the invading presence of his estranged half-brother, Albert.

'We're not talking about boys and girls anymore,' Albert said after fixing himself a Dewar's straight up. 'We're talking about harsh metaphysical realities, resounding eternal conflicts of the inalienable human spirit, wild powers set loose in the night. Dark, primitive forces, Roland. I told you to *negate* women. I never meant you could just *ignore* them.'

'I'm not trying to negate or ignore anybody,' Roland said simply. 'I just want to be alone and hear myself think.' He was sitting in his easy chair, growing slowly aware of a vast, unsettling stillness in the streets outside. No footsteps, no whispers. No hum or charge of the cold moon.

Albert noticed it too.

'Hear that, Roland? Do you *hear* that?' Albert gestured with his Dewar's at the intense implacable absence of it all. Anti-everything. Unthinkability. Non-being. Non-to-be and non-ever-been. 'You can't *ignore* physics, bro. You can't run off and disavow energy, or gravity, or life. You've taken negativity a step too far and turned it into something else. If you negate the negator, Roland, what have you got? You remember your bonehead algebra, don't you? Put two negatives together and what's the product?'

'A positive,' Roland said meekly. Far in the distance, a wind was beginning to rise. Sweeping dead leaves through the streets. Rattling the high power and telephone lines.

'That's right, bro. Negate the negator and you've got a

positive, right? But if you try to negate *negating* the negator? Are you following me, bro? What have you got *then*?'

'Negativity,' Roland said. His confusion felt like clarity. In not understanding, he finally seemed to understand. 'Pure negativity and nothing else.'

'You've created a philosophical conundrum, bro. It's what I call a "desire displacement vortex." You've negated all these terrific babes, but you haven't given them anything to negate in return. So they're out there rushing around. All restless with desire to be someplace other than they already are. It's not sexual dynamics anymore, Roland. It's bigger than that. It's bigger than you and me put together.'

As it approached the house, Roland realized it wasn't wind anymore. It wasn't storm, or force, or echo. It wasn't a lot of things. In many ways, it wasn't even out there.

The windows began to shudder in their windowframes. The doors began to chatter.

Albert swallowed the last of his Dewar's just before the glass in his hand shattered from a high-pitched keening sound.

'Oh hell,' Albert said, and picked a fragment of glass from his lower lip. He looked at Roland. 'I tried to warn you, bro.'

The entire house began to rumble. Roland's ears and sinuses filled with pressure as if he were descending in an airplane.

'There's just one part I don't understand!' Roland shouted. He tried to stand from his chair. The noise was lifting through the floorboards. Suddenly the entire house was thundering with it.

'Are they doing this because they *like* us?' Roland cried. 'Or is it because they *don't* like us at all?'

Albert was squinting through a rain of crumbling plaster. Behind him, a bookshelf toppled. A painting fell off the wall.

'What's that, bro?' Albert shouted. 'I can't hear you!'

But by this point, nobody could hear anything.

believe me

michael carson

Forgive me, Father. I didn't mean to startle you. Mind you, the sudden way you turned and the look you gave me quite undid me for a moment there – I, who should be well past further undoing by now. Would it come as a surprise if I were to tell you that even I am capable of being shocked? You wouldn't believe me for a moment, would you? No, I thought not. I am seldom believed even when I speak true. But believe me when I tell you – for what possible advantage might I gain from a lie? Are you not already mine? – that I have not come to you today in order to gloat. That would be too cruel, and I am not without sentiment, Father Keogh.

Here you sit, Father, on a grubby corporation bench, gazing out at the brown winter estuary. There aren't many ships going up and down the river to Liverpool, are there? Not like when you were a boy. Not like when you sailed out, your head set fair towards sanctity, all those years ago on one of those ubiquitous The-British-Are-Coming Blue Funnel ships. The Mersey's gone to the devil and no mistake.

I wish I could show you a couple of snapshots of yourself. A waving 'then' and a wan 'now'. But I don't need to, do I? You know exactly what you look like, can take in the whole situation even through those tears you're shedding. (You've got a drop on the end of your nose by the way.) Is it always like this?

Yes, you know this picture. Before you walked into it hopeless a few minutes ago you had conjured it up a million times. On every occasion that I attempted to make you give up your work at the Muru Mission, planting in your brain optimistic pictures of loved ones back home and sunsets and snowfalls and sandhills and ship-spotting and spring-boarding into the depths of the New Brighton baths; commanding all the uncomfortable things I had at my disposal in paradisal Muru: mosquitos and bureaucrats and thorns and leeches and tourists and, of course, your little failing, in your direction . . . you would imagine yourself here on such a dead day as this, back where you had begun, a stranger to home, a man old and unsung, cold in the stone wind blowing in this dog-squatting, paint-sprayed, old-joke jerk of the atlas that you cannot catechize and do not understand. And the picture was enough to nullify all nostalgia, to pour balm on your bites and render useless all my hard work.

Don't look at me like that! Honestly, anyone would think I was just trying to make matters worse. Believe me, such is not the case. I do pity you, Father Keogh. No, really. To tell you the truth, I cannot wait to be off to warmer climes. You know, I just may return to the mission to see how everything is working out. Yes, I'll maybe pop in on – I forget his name – your servant of thirty years. Ah, yes. Anselm. Thank you. I was greatly moved by the single chaste kiss you placed upon Anselm's furrowed brown forehead before you descended into the dugout, blessed your flock in your practised priestly manner and then watched them serenely as they sang 'The Ship of Faith', your fragile vessel paddling you out of their lives on your way back to this place. Yes, I may well return. I wonder what Anselm is thinking? Do you know, Father? I rather think he does not know whether he is coming or going.

Coming and going! I have made a joke. A laugh, I suppose, is too much to expect. But not even a wry smile, Father!

No. Even that is too much, I suppose.

Let me give you a bit of advice. A sense of humour might yet save you. Believe it or not. I can even be that frank without fear that you will take me seriously. You feel so safe in your seriousness, just as you once felt safe in your worthiness.

Ah, I wonder what has become of all those devoted golden girls you seduced into covering their charms, keeping their virtue, hiding their nether endowments? Are they as we speak – or rather as I speak, for you are at long last past speech – gathered round the harmonium in the rattan chapel lustily singing out 'What Have I Done For My God Today?' Do they, I wonder, feel the lack of a priest? Perhaps the feeling of being so long restrained has become irksome and they are loosening their sweaty Christian clothing. A button opened here. A strap let fall there. Eyes a little less blinkered, on the look out for the forbidden fruit of young men with flowers behind their ears, slim brown bodies in paradisal sarongs poling up the shallows surrounded by parrots and lilies and low mist. Who knows, Father, perhaps even your dear Anselm has become an object of desire for them.

It was, I have to admit, a master stroke on my part to have the government decide that no further visas would be issued to clerics once you had – how shall I put it? – gone. It took a fair leap in lateral thinking to arrange that, you know. The pious Muslim shopkeeper, Ali Mohammed, depended on the mission's custom for his livelihood as surely as you and your flock depended on him for your necessities. I would not have thought it possible a mere year ago that he would have sacrificed prosperity for the sake of principle. It's odd how things work out.

I planted the thought in his head when he was at his strongest and, therefore, his weakest.

Ali Mohammed was on the flight back from the Haj. I caught sight of him refusing the proffered meal, concentrating instead on reading inspirational literature. Now's my chance, I thought. He came to a point in the pamphlet which exhorted the good Haji to sacrifice all for righteousness's sake. As he placed his right thumb between the leaves as a bookmark, closing his eyes the better to meditate on the text as the jet engines roared outside, I whispered to him in that way I have. *Haji Ali Mohammed, you are the strongest pillar of Islam on the Muru river yet you allow, perhaps even encourage, the mission. Now I know The Prophet preached tolerance, but enough is enough. Would it not be heroic of you to put in a word with your devout and powerful friends in The Capital . . . a word about priests . . .* Then I watched him for a moment, admiring the way he had got his moustaches to curl so spectacularly. Mine, though I have tried for ages, do not hold a candle to his. But that is by the by.

There was no immediate effect and off I went to see if I could justify the devilish expense of the flight with a few minor achievements. A steward was asking a young Haji if he would like wine with his meal. I noted the look of affront on the young man's face and beamed him a strong temptation, stronger than – looking back – was fair in the circumstances. *Yes, please*, he said. I stayed around until the wine arrived and he had quaffed part of it. I noted the look of youth and hope drain from his face.

Towards the back of the plane – I always find the smoking section an excellent setting for my work – I started an argument between a couple who had been married for twenty years and had not had a cross word in all that time. I made the man think some thoughts about his wife which he had buried deep. He spoke them in the heat of the moment and she started to cry. Her mascara dripped black down her face. He looked at her and told her she was old and ugly. Well satisfied, I drifted back to Haji. He seemed just as I had left him, though his thoughts were going hay-wire. Do you know what he was thinking, Father Keogh? I blush to tell you. Haji had it in mind to tell the religious authorities that all priests should be expelled from The Republic immediately! All mission stations were to be taken over by the government and the area colonized by Muslim bachelors from that overcrowded island where even I don't dare set foot! Well, you can imagine my reaction to that!

No, I see you can't. How very far you are from understanding my ways! I was against such draconian methods and I will tell you for why. Humans are always tempted by the most extreme paths. You all love the Water Cannon. I go for the slow torture of the dripping tap. Long experience has taught me that a drip of forgetfulness here, a drop of neglect there, a pool of rancour over there, is much more effective than a fountain or a flood.

But back to Haji. All I did was whisper that he need not embark on such an extreme course of action. He had to nurture his little piece of venture capital, after all. He might, however, drop a word in the right ear about visas. Of course, I thought that once he got home and mused on the practicalities of life and the necessity of earning a living, his good intentions would go sailing down the river like the Coke cans and cardboard packing cases he never tires of dumping in it. I forgot about him and turned my attention back to you.

You! How holy you were growing! You were beginning to be seen as a saint in your own lifetime. Your fame had spread as far as the headwaters of the Muru and into the massif beyond. People paddled for days to be swaddled by your shadow. Father Keogh who heals with a touch, with a pill, with a prick, with a nonchalant gesture of his hand. Holy Keogh.

The trouble was that you believed it – stop me if I am being uncharitable – you believed in your holiness yourself. Not all the time of course, and you fought the feeling whenever it

bubbled up into consciousness. But in your subconscious –
where all the really interesting stuff goes on and where I set up
my bivouac – you were secure in your utter worthiness. It
drove the angels nuts, I can tell you. Me, I just smiled.

You see, with the passing of years your growing perception
of your own worthiness gave me the chink into which I could
insert my little lever that neatly flicks worlds over. You had
forgotten about Anselm, hadn't you? Poor Anselm! Hand-
picked by young Father Keogh long before the blotting-paper
of piety had completely dried up your lust, before your
heaven-gazing eye had seen through the attractions of a well-
turned limb, a sunshine smile, a soil-and-water-spangled
physique.

So see young Anselm see-saw in his sarong of many
colours. You relieved him of his sarong and in its place kitted
him out in khaki and a Sunday best of surplus and cotta. But
in those first years, when your sap was singing, you taught
him things his people had never dreamed of. You took his
head and turned it where it would succour you. And then
later you told him to turn his face to the front again, to blot
out from his young mind what had occurred, to shut his fair
lips against all shame, to fix his thoughts on the old rugged
cross.

I am well aware that I am twisting the dagger that has
already taken your life but I really feel it to be necessary.
Believe me, this hurts me as well as you. Anselm was your sin.
He is the reason you sit here now, collapsed. But he was not
your sin in the way you think. Your youthful coupling could
have passed unnoticed.

Oh, how slow you are! You do not perceive it even now.
You think that you have sinned, shrived him, left him whole.
It was all so long ago. You imagine that now he is managing to
captain a little Christian barque in a Muslim and Animist sea.
Deprived of a priest the Muru mission may be, but it has

Anselm, your loyal and chaste deacon, to help it foghorn through the encircling gloom.

I believe, however, that you are mistaken. Anselm is as split as The Trinity. One man containing a childhood of forest and river spirits, the life-in-death gospel story and . . . what is the third part? Not Islam. I think he will resist it. No, the third part of Anselm is the desire you awoke in him and then – when remorse and a certain slackening of the heart's desire hit you – tried to root out. The lad did not know any more who he was. He still does not. What, stiff with longing, you referred to as *brotherly love* and then, when he had knelt to show Father how much he cared and made a good job of it, you, detumescent and depressed, got down beside him on your knees to pray forgiveness for . . . that has become part of Anselm.

I dwell on Anselm because it seems to me that he is a potent metaphor for what you missionaries do. You split asunder. You set father against son. You draw ruled borders up and down and across brains, and in the little square warring countries of the mind thus created you write sums that do not add up.

But I do not blame you alone, Father Keogh. The chastity enjoined upon the anointed in your brand of religion! It has given us from the infernal regions a splendid time over the aeons. Now, I'm not against chastity per se. Perish the thought. Doubtless there are some whom it suits. But when I think of the clients I've had who have come over to me because of the chaste clergy, I have to wonder. In my book it would be fine if it were only the priests and religious who paid for their lack of fleshly companionship, but experience teaches me otherwise. Everyone the holding-back cleric approaches pays dearly. The classroom cuff that is loaded with last night's struggle against forbidden longings; the confessional tirade longer and louder because the poor confessor lusts for the sin himself; the catechisms of impossible difficulty framed by dithery celibates to make the ordinary chap stumble over scruples. It was, dear Father Keogh, your flock who paid the price for the public virtue of the lonely shepherd. The bad shepherd fucks his sheep. Either that or he fucks them up, whets their appetite for the strange taste of the yew tree.

How angry you were when you discovered the bag of love herbs hanging round Anselm's neck, along with the crucifix you had given him long years before. You ripped the bag off and threw it in the river, telling him how disappointed you were that after all those years he had returned to his wicked ways. But those charms were his upbringing, Father Keogh, just as surely as medals, rosaries and missals were yours. The elders of his village were as appalled by his crucifix as you were by his charms.

His charms! Ha!

What is truth? No doubt you'll be shocked but I have a certain regard for Pontius Pilate. But, had Pilate never ventured abroad, never seen the stiff-necked monotheism of the Jews, he would not have asked such a cynical question. Truth would have been as clear as the nose on the emperor's face. His question was the mark of the split man. And, as I have said before, into the split goes the devil's lever.

And the truth of Anselm? When you stopped pleading for his youthful favours poor Anselm was already split. For years, when you thought he was away on mission business, Anselm was taking care of his own. I knew that, of course. I often accompanied him. I piloted him, you might say. We left you behind at the mission, wrapped up in your work and your worthiness. Had you not managed to put the devil of desire to death?

But sins will find you out. They live on in those you have offended. It only remained for me – being as you must know by now a shameful gossip – to whisper my suspicions into Haji's ears. Haji was ready, primed for economic martyrdom. Did he know, I said, that wicked Father Keogh had caused poor Anselm to become habituated in vice? Could he not, by having a shameless surrogate ply Anselm with liquor while in one of the sinks of The Capital, hear the whole sorry story?

And Anselm, drunk and bereft, told his tale to an eager listener. To the hearer it was a garment-ripping story of lust and unnatural passion; to Anselm one of unrequited love, the highpoint of his low life. Rending his garments, Haji's messenger returned with the story that had you expelled.

It's all quite simple. The Order thinks you are *recovering* among friends and family. They are even thinking of sending you to the mission-fields of South America; have – if my intelligence is correct – arranged for a Spanish Linguaphone course to be hand-delivered to you by T.N.T. They do not realize that you are lost. You feel you deserve debasement, everything you are feeling now. You cannot forgive yourself. You have returned to find Liverpool a theme park, the swimming pool you so loved filled in and covered over with greensward – likewise the people you loved, the people who thought your holy work would pull them into paradise.

It's all changed, just as you changed everything at the mission. I shall always remember the people of the Muru mission. It's probably not my place to say, but they were so Christlike until you found them and pushed them into the rule-tattooed arms of an angry God. I feel sorry for them, believe me. And I remember the bag of charms you ripped from Anselm's neck. Do you know what they were for, Father Keogh? They were concocted in order to rekindle your dead heart. Well, that's all down the river now. The herbs and butterfly wings and bird-feathers and little chameleon bones and Anselm's spittle and a hair taken from your bed, are so much scum on the waters of another river far away.

Hey, look, Father Keogh! Through the swirling fog along the promenade, his head lowered against the wicked wind, walks a young man. From the look of him he has just ripped open the promising package of his twenties. Here he comes. Not bad, eh? Why not? No harm in trying. It's perfectly legal. Ask him the time. Be sure, Father Keogh, he's past corruption. See the leylines of life on his young face. No harm will come of it, believe me. And what do you have to lose?

Nothing.

Believe me.

choosing
the incubus

molly brown

'Vivid dreams of a sexual nature?' the doctor repeated, nodding thoughtfully. He smiled at the twenty-something, red-haired woman sitting on the other side of his desk. 'Lucky you. How long has this been going on?'

'About three weeks. Ever since I moved into my new flat.'

He leaned back, making a steeple with his hands. 'Well, that explains it. Moving house is always stressful – these dreams are merely your subconscious's way of dealing with stress. And a jolly nice way of dealing with it, too.'

'What about the scratches? The teeth marks?'

'You did those yourself. You'd be amazed what people can get up to in their sleep.' He looked down, breaking their eye contact, and busied himself with separating the stack of papers on his desk into separate, equal piles. 'Good day, Miss Baker. I have patients with *real* problems waiting to see me.'

That night it happened again. Kisses. Deep, luscious kisses. Coral opened her mouth, responding to the tongue that gently probed; she moaned with pleasure as the tongue explored the rest of her body. The probing became harder; more insistent. A weight pushed down upon her, and her moans became screams of ecstasy.

Catlike, she stretched in the morning sun, her eyes still closed from sleep, her lips turned up in a satisfied grin. She

rolled over, reached out, and wrapped her arms around –
nothing.

'Oh no,' she said out loud to an empty room, 'not again.
Please not again!'

Gerald phoned from Vienna that afternoon; his seminar on
'Accountancy in a United Europe' was over and he'd be flying
back that evening. This weekend it would be his place.

She was in Gerald's kitchen when he opened his front door
and set down his suitcase. 'What's for dinner?' he said.

Later that night, moving on top of her, he whispered,
'Vienna is an . . . amazingly . . . beautiful city . . . mmm, you
would . . . have . . . ,' his voice raised to a shout, 'uh! uh! uh!
Aaaaah . . . loved the buildings.' He rolled on to his back and
lit a cigarette. 'And the food! Those pastries!'

'Hmmm?' Coral said.

They spent most of Saturday out on the balcony. Gerald
spent the day working on his seminar report for the other
department heads. Coral read a book. After dinner, Gerald
fondled her breasts and told her how the other departments
were due for a real shake-up. 'Ooh, baby,' Gerald said before
falling asleep.

She didn't want to go home alone on Sunday, but Gerald
reminded her of their agreement that career came first. They
never spent the night together when there was work in the
morning. Gerald kissed her on the cheek and told her he'd see
her next Friday at her place.

Coral's flesh rose up in tiny bumps the minute she walked
into her flat. It was the middle of August; there was no reason
why the place should be so cold. She walked into her bedroom
and it was *freezing*. She turned on the heat and started to get
undressed. Slipping out of her jeans, she felt strangely self-
conscious, as if she wasn't alone. She put her jeans back on.

Armed with a knife from the kitchen, she searched every

corner. Satisfied that she was alone and that every door and window was locked securely, she went to bed fully dressed.

The next morning, she found her jeans on the floor.

I did that myself, she thought. I was uncomfortable and I took them off. That's all there is to it. *I did that myself*, she thought over and over.

She'd drunk six cups of coffee and was on her fifteenth cigarette when there was a knock on her office door. She jumped. 'Who is it?'

The door opened and Abby, who had the office next door, marched in. Fifty, fat, and twice-divorced, she had been Coral's self-appointed protector, adviser, and surrogate mother-figure since the younger woman's first day on the job, a situation which Coral sometimes found annoying, but had come to accept.

Abby stopped in front of Coral's desk, folded her arms across her chest, and glared. 'Well? Are you going to tell me what's wrong?'

'I . . . I don't know what you mean.'

'I thought we were friends, Coral. Friends talk to each other. They tell each other when something's wrong.'

'There's nothing wrong.'

'Nothing wrong? You've been holed up in your office all week, and if anybody so much as looks at you, you jump a mile!'

'No, I don't,' Coral said quickly.

'Ha!' said Abby, 'pull the other one! What about yesterday? Poor old Henderson only had to say "good morning" to make you knock over a stack of files. And the day before that, when you spilled coffee all over those computer disks? And . . .'

Coral raised a hand to stop her. 'Okay, okay. Point taken. Maybe I'm a little tense, but it's nothing, really. I just haven't been getting enough sleep lately, that's all.'

Abby's expression changed to a mischievous grin. 'Don't tell me you finally dumped that horrible twerp and got yourself a real man? About time, girl!'

Coral's face turned red.

'That's it, isn't it?' Abby went on, deliberately misinterpreting Coral's reaction. She leaned forward, lowering her voice to a husky, suggestive whisper. 'No one ever gets a wink of sleep for those first few weeks, do they? Who is he? Do I know him? Not that it matters – anything's better than that last one of yours; I don't know what you ever saw in him.'

Coral bit her lip, fuming. 'You've made it quite clear you don't like him, but Gerald has many fine qualities of which you are obviously unaware,' she said, struggling to keep her voice under control. 'He's . . . reliable. And stable . . . and honest, and . . . reliable. And if you had any idea how many two-faced bastards I've had to put up with in the past,' her eyes began to fill with tears, 'you'd realize just how important reliable is!' The tears were spilling down her cheeks. 'Oh, damn!' She angrily wiped her face with the back of one hand.

'I'm sorry!' Abby looked around the room in desperation. 'I'd offer you a tissue, but I can't find one! Where do you keep them?'

'Here.' Coral reached into a desk drawer and pulled one out, loudly blowing her nose.

'Look, I'm really sorry,' Abby repeated. 'I was way out of line, talking about your boyfriend like that. I didn't mean it, love. Honest. I was only winding you up – I never thought you'd take me seriously. You know what a kidder I am! I like Gerald. He's a great bloke, really. And he makes you very happy – anyone can see that.'

'Yes, he does,' Coral agreed, sobbing.

Abby hesitated a moment before saying, 'This doesn't mean lunch is off, does it?'

The weekend was a disaster. Coral couldn't relax in bed; she felt they were being watched. She nearly screamed for Gerald to stop – the room around them had come to life, watching with glowing red eyes, throbbing with jealous desire – but before she could say anything, he was already lying spent beside her, breathing softly with his head on her shoulder. Six months ago – even two or three weeks ago – she might have looked at him tenderly, or even kissed his forehead. He was good-looking, he had a well-paid job and a lot of ambition, and as far as she knew, he'd never cheated on her. That had been enough for her once. Now she just wanted him to leave. She wanted to be alone, to surrender herself, alone, to the feeling that permeated the room.

She lay there seething with frustration as Gerald snored beside her. She slid one hand along her inner thigh, moving upwards, and then she stopped, embarrassed. She was being watched; she *knew* she was being watched.

She slept all day Saturday. When she woke up that evening, Gerald told her he'd had a productive day; he'd brought his lap-top computer with him.

Later that night, Coral's bedroom pulsated with anger and indignation. Gerald didn't notice. He climbed on top of Coral, and she rolled her eyes, grimacing in the dark.

When Gerald left on Sunday evening, Coral breathed a sigh of relief. She rushed into the bathroom and lathered herself with perfumed soap. She lingered in the shower, revelling in the way the water pounded against her skin. Then she got into bed and she waited.

By the middle of the week, everyone at work noticed that Coral seemed to be her old self again. In fact, they'd never seen her so happy – no one had ever seen her giggle over a group pension plan before.

She knocked on Abby's office door and offered to treat her to lunch.

'So what's all this about?' Abby asked, looking around the expensive restaurant Coral had taken her to. A uniformed waiter poured them each a glass of champagne.

'I'm celebrating.'

'Celebrating what?'

'The fact that I've finally managed to accept something.'

'And what have you accepted?'

Coral shrugged and raised her glass in a toast. 'The fact that I've gone crazy. Stark staring mad. Bonkers. Utterly ga-ga.'

'What?'

'I'm afraid so. I'm totally insane.'

'You must be, ordering champagne on your salary.'

'Oh, it's not just that. It's things that have been happening. Fun things. Things that happen late at night, when I think I'm all alone, but I'm not . . . Or I think I'm awake, but I'm not. Oh here comes the food. Thank goodness, I'm starving.'

'Fun things?' Abby repeated, starting to giggle. 'Fun how?'

Coral told her. A man at the next table leaned so far over he fell off his chair.

Coral was wakened by the passionate mouth that forced her lips apart, giving access to that long and insistent tongue that she had come to know so well. She let out a groan of pleasure as her legs parted and the thrusting began.

She was awake. Though her eyes were still closed, she was definitely awake and she was being made love to. The weight that pressed upon her, moving in rhythmic waves, was real. There was no doubt about it. She could hear moans so loud they bounced off the walls, and they weren't all coming from her. Her body began to spasm, over and over again. She cried out and dug her nails deep into something above her. Something solid. Something that didn't feel right.

Gasping for breath, she opened her eyes. More than anything in the world, she wanted to run. She wanted to scream and scream until her throat had torn itself to shreds. She wanted to fall down on her knees and pray.

She didn't do any of these things because she fainted.

The alarm clock went off at seven. She reached over to shut it off and lay there for a moment, feeling drained. Her eyelids fluttered open and she stared up at the ceiling. Then she remembered. There was no time for a shower or make-up, she had to get out of there. She leaped out of bed, threw on some clothes with awkward, shaking hands, and ran out the door.

She phoned Gerald from a coin box. His voice was gruff and sleepy. No, he couldn't possibly take the day off. There was an important meeting that morning and he had to be there. He'd see her tomorrow, anyway, so what was the problem? Oh yes, he added, he might have a surprise for her. His alarm clock rang, and he hung up.

It was seven-fifteen in the morning and she had no family and very few friends. There was nobody she could run to; there was no place she could go except to work. She walked in circles for an hour and then she spent twenty minutes waiting outside the front door because she'd forgotten her key. She threw up in the toilet across from her office.

That afternoon, she knocked on Abby's office door.

'Coral? What are you still doing here? I thought you went home ill.'

Coral sat down across from Abby. 'I have been ill. But I didn't go home. I couldn't go home . . .' She leaned forward, resting both her elbows on Abby's desk. She lowered her voice. 'You remember those dreams I told you about?'

Abby laughed. 'How could I forget?'

'They weren't dreams!' Coral leaned even further forward. 'Do you know what an incubus is?'

'A what?'

'It's a demon. A male demon who has sex with mortal women.'

'Coral, stop it right now. You sound positively medieval!'

'That's exactly it! In the Middle Ages, women who had sex with demons were burned at the stake.'

'That was just superstition; there's no such thing as a demon.'

'That's what I thought. But then I saw one. It's got burning red eyes, and leather wings, just like a bat. And it was in my bed!'

Abby nodded slowly, a tight little smile on her face. 'Sure, Coral.'

'Don't humour me, Abby! I remember reading about it at university, in a book about witch-trials in the Middle Ages. According to this book, in the fourteenth century, several unmarried women in a particular village gave birth to deformed children with wings! The women were tried for witchcraft and each confessed that she'd had sex with a demon, who she now realized had only been using her to reproduce its kind upon the earth. They all said the same thing: that a creature with black wings and eyes like burning coals had come to them in the night, every night. Sometimes several times a night. But the most important thing is this: after the women were tried and found guilty, the village they lived in was deserted – no one would live there any more. They thought the place itself was evil. And you know where that place is? Exactly where I'm living now!'

Abby raised one eyebrow. 'In your flat? Stop winding me up.'

'On that *land*. My flat's in a new development – I'm sure it's the same place because the land was empty until the developer bought it. It's been empty for hundreds of years. They were afraid to build anything there after what happened, don't you see?'

Abby thought for a moment before speaking very slowly and carefully. 'Is there something you're unhappy about, Coral?'

'Something I'm unhappy about?' Coral repeated incredulously. She stood up, staring at Abby in wide-eyed amazement. 'Of course there is! I'm unhappy there's a sex-mad demon in my flat! Wouldn't you be?'

'That's not what I meant,' Abby said. 'I mean, could there be something that on a conscious level, you don't want to face? Something you're pushing so far down inside you, that your subconscious decides it's got to *make* you face whatever it is – this problem you're denying – and the only way your subconscious can do it is to conjure up some image from your past, like this demon from a book you once read?'

Oh *no*, Coral thought, she's read something in *Woman's Weekly* and now she's an expert. 'No,' she said, shaking her head. 'No, there's nothing.'

'You're sure?'

'Of course I'm sure!'

'Coral, I'm no psychiatrist or anything . . .'

'But I thought you were,' Coral interrupted sarcastically.

'All I'm trying to say is if you think about it, doesn't this demon of yours sound just a little bit Freudian?'

Coral brought her fist down on the desk. 'I'm telling you there is something in my flat – not a dream, not a subconscious symbol – something one hundred per cent real and very, very physical!'

Abby leaned back and sighed. 'I suppose you'd better come and stay at my place.'

Coral arrived at Gerald's flat only a few minutes ahead of him. 'I haven't had time to start the dinner – I only just got here.'

'That's okay,' he told her. 'I was going to take you out for dinner, anyway.'

Her jaw dropped in surprise. They *never* went out to dinner; Gerald always said there was nothing like good home cooking. 'Really?'

He smiled at her reaction, and it struck her that he always looked so smug. 'Really,' he said.

After they handed their menus back to the waiter, Coral looked across the candlelit table and asked if this was the surprise he'd mentioned yesterday morning.

He shook his head. 'I got my place on the Board. Sooner than I expected.'

'Oh, Gerald, that's wonderful! You've been wanting that so badly.'

'I know. And now there's something else I want. To make my life complete.' He reached across and took her hand.

'And what's that, Gerald?'

'Children.'

'WHAT?'

'I've been thinking about this for a while, Coral. Of course I didn't want to say anything until I was certain. But now, with this promotion, I think the time has come.'

'Has it?'

'It has. Oh, we'll get married of course. And as soon as property starts looking up again, we can sell your flat and get a house in Sussex, near the Downs. It'll be great for the kids.'

'Kids,' Coral repeated. 'That's a plural.'

'I want at least four. Two boys, two girls.'

'You realize this could make things a bit difficult for me at work, don't you?'

Gerald chuckled politely and squeezed her hand in appreciation. 'You've always had such a sense of humour. Of course you'll quit your job. Being a wife and mother is work enough for any woman.'

'But I've moved up very fast. I could be assistant district manager when Mr Henderson retires.'

'Tut-tut, darling. You know you'll never get as far or make as much money as I will, so why bother trying? Of course, I'll let you keep working long enough to get some paid maternity leave . . .'

That night, Gerald asked her if she'd taken her pill and she said yes. Oh well, he told her, you can forget about those darn things as of tomorrow. She closed her eyes.

'Mmm, baby, baby,' he said, pressing down on her in the dark.

'You're crushing my leg.'

'Sorry.' He shifted his weight.

'Not that one, the other one.'

He moved again.

'Mind my . . . ow!'

'Now what's wrong?'

'You're pulling my hair!'

'Sorry.'

He grunted, sighed, muttered something about re-joining the exchange-rate mechanism, and went to sleep. She got up and took a long, hot bath, remembering the way every nerve-end had tingled with exquisite sensation only two nights earlier. Then she visualized herself, five years down the road, living with Gerald and Gerald's children, and never feeling that way again.

Saturday morning, she asked him if he enjoyed having sex with her. 'What a stupid question,' he said, patting her on the hand.

They spent the afternoon on the balcony and he told her what a great life they were going to have out in the country where there would be nothing to distract her from the joy of presiding over a brood of miniature Geralds. With the approach of evening, Coral noticed how the red light of the sunset reflected in his eyes, making them glow like a pair of hot coals. She couldn't stop herself imagining him with a pair of leather wings.

'You want to use me to reproduce your kind upon the earth, don't you?' she said.

He looked surprised for a moment, and then he smiled. 'Well, I could hardly manage it without you, could I?'

She swallowed her pill when he wasn't looking.

'Fingers crossed,' Gerald said later, doing a flying leap on to the mattress which broke the bedframe, throwing splinters in all directions.

On Sunday, for the first time ever, he told her that she didn't have to leave. 'I can drive over and pick up the rest of your clothes,' he offered, sitting on the mattress which now rested on the floor.

'No, Gerald,' she told him. 'I want to go home.'

'Okay,' he said. 'We'll go to your place. This making a baby business does take a bit of effort, but I think I'm up to another go.'

'No, please. I don't think my furniture could take the strain.'

Her phone rang at eleven o'clock. It was Abby. 'Are you all right? I thought you were coming back here tonight.'

'I'm fine. And I don't think I'll be needing your hospitality after all. I'm going to stay right here.'

'But . . . but you said there was an evil spirit in your flat that wanted to use you to reproduce its kind upon the earth.'

'Did I say that? I must have been winding you up. Well, never mind. Everything's all right now. There's no problem . . .

no problem at all.' She put down the phone and turned off the light.

She lay alone in the darkness, giggling. That poor little demon from the fourteenth century would never have heard of birth control.

about the authors

Lisa Appignanesi's novels include *Memory and Desire* (1991) and *Dreams of Innocence* (1994). She is also the co-author of *Freud's Women* (1992) with John Forrester and she has produced a number of television films.

Scott Bradfield was born in San Francisco and now divides his time between London and the University of Connecticut, where he is Assistant Professor of English. He is the author of a novel, *The History of Luminous Motion*; a collection of short stories, *Greetings from Earth*; and a study of American literature, *Dreaming Revolution: Transgression in the Development of American Romance*. His new novel, *What's Wrong with America*, will be published in 1994.

Ian Breakwell exhibits regularly at Anthony Reynolds Gallery in London. His artworks hang in public collections, including the Tate Gallery. His books include *The Artist's Dream*, *Seeing in the Dark: A Compendium of Cinemagoing* (co-edited with Paul Hammond) and *Ian Breakwell's Diary*, which has been serialized on both radio and television. He has recently had exhibitions in Cardiff, Southampton, and at the Victoria and Albert Museum and the ICA in London.

Molly Brown has been everything from an armed guard to the voice of a cartoon bear. She has had a number of stories published in the crime, science fiction and fantasy genres, and won the British Science Fiction Award for the Best Short Story of 1991.

Michael Carson taught English as a foreign language around the world for fifteen years, but now lives in Powys. He has published many successful novels, including *Sucking Sherbet Lemons* and *Yanking Up the Yo-Yo*, and a book of short stories, *Serving Suggestions*.

Matt Cohen was born in Kingston, Ontario. He has since spent several years in England and France, as well as teaching at various Canadian universities. His novels include *The Spanish Doctor*, *Nadine*, *Emotional Arithmetic* and *The Bookseller*. His short story collections are *The Expatriate*, *Café le Dog* and *Living on Water*.

Evelyn Conlon lives in Dublin. She is the author of a novel, *Stars in the Daytime*, and two collections of short stories, *My Head is Opening* and *Taking Scarlet as a Real Colour*.

Jane DeLynn is the author of the novels, *Some Do*, *In Thrall*, *Real Estate* and *Don Juan in the Village*. She has also published a number of short stories and articles for such publications as *Rolling Stone*, *The New York Times Magazine*, *Harper's Bazaar* and *Mademoiselle*. She lives in New York.

Alison Fell is a Scottish poet and novelist who lives in London. She has published four novels, two collections of poetry and several women's anthologies. Her novel *Mer de Glace* won the Boardman Tasker Award for Mountain Literature.

Victor Headley's first novel, *Yardie*, topped the London bestseller charts for three months in the summer of 1992. The sequel, *Excess*, was published in 1993. He lives in Hackney.

Catherine Hiller is the author of the novels *An Old Friend from High School*, *17 Morton Street* and *California Time*. She has won two PEN Syndicated Fiction Awards and teaches novel-writing at the Writer's Voice in New York City. She is the producer of the documentary films, *Do Not Enter: The Visa War Against Ideas* and *Paul Bowles: The Complete Outsider*. She lives in Mamaroneck, NY.

Christopher Hope was born in South Africa but has lived in England since 1975. His most recent book is a collection of linked tales, *The Love Songs of Nathan J. Swirsky*, published in 1993.

John Hoyland lives in London and works for *New Scientist*. He has published a children's novel, *The Ivy Garland*, is co-author with Jonathan Chadwick of two plays, and is the editor of *Fathers and Sons*, published by Serpent's Tail.

Eroica Mildmay grew up in West and North Africa. She studied art and has worked as a fashion model and in the film business. Her first novel, *Lucker and Tiffany Peel Out*, was published by Serpent's Tail in 1993.

Jill Neville arrived in London from Australia at the age of eighteen and has remained there, except for six years based in Paris and four years back in Sydney. Her sixth novel, *Swimming the Channel*, was published in 1992.

Sean O Caoimh lives in Paris and Provence. France is an antidote to his Irish childhood, English education and prolonged exposure to the American mercantile culture. He reads mid-European literature and occasionally pokes the embers and tries to fan into small flames the combustions of his own past. These slippery images he converts into poetry and short stories, some of which are published in obscure literary magazines. He likes wood sailing vessels and wantons. He dislikes mannered, *passionless* English fiction.

Joseph O'Connor was born in Dublin in 1963. His debut novel, *Cowboys and Indians*, was shortlisted for the Whitbread Prize and his first collection of short stories, *True Believers*, received widespread critical acclaim. His second novel, *Desperadoes*, will be published in 1994. He has written film and television scripts, journalism and a biography of the Irish poet, Charles Donnelly, *Even the Olives Are Bleeding*. He has won the Hennessy New Irish Writer of the Year Award, the *Time Out* Travel Writing Prize and the 1993 Macaulay Fellowship of the Irish Arts Council/*An Chomhairle Ealaíon*.

Marge Piercy is the author of twelve collections of poetry, a book of craft essays and twelve novels, including *Woman on the Edge of Time*, *Vida*, *Braided Lives*, *Gone to Soldiers*, *Summer People* and *Body of Glass*, which won the Arthur C. Clarke Award for Best Science Fiction Published in the United Kingdom in 1992. She is the poetry editor of *Tikkun* and her fiction and poetry have been translated into fourteen languages. She lives in Wellfleet on Cape Cod.

Kate Pullinger comes from Canada but has lived in Britain since 1982. Her novels are *Tiny Lies*, *When the Monster Dies* and *Where Does Kissing End?* She has edited *A Gambling Box* and an anthology of short stories, *Border Lines*. She is Fellow in Creative Writing at the University of Reading and Visiting Writer at the Newport Gwent School of Art and Design. She lives in London.

Christopher Rawlence is a writer, a film-maker and librettist. His books include *About Time* and *The Missing Reel*; his librettos *The Man Who Mistook His Wife for a Hat* and *King of Hearts*. He has made many television films and lives in London.

Mary Scott is the author of *Nudists May be Encountered* and *Not in Newbury*, both published by Serpent's Tail. She has written short stories for anthologies, magazines and Radio 4; contributed to *Guardian Woman*; and is books editor for *Everywoman*. She lives in London.